Fayçal Zeroual

CLINICAL EXAMINATION OF THE COW'S GENITAL TRACT

Fayçal Zeroual

CLINICAL EXAMINATION OF THE COW'S GENITAL TRACT

ScienciaScripts

Imprint

Cover image: www.ingimage.com

This book is a translation from the original published under ISBN 978-620-6-70627-4.

Publisher:
Sciencia Scripts
is a trademark of
Dodo Books Indian Ocean Ltd. and OmniScriptum S.R.L publishing group

120 High Road, East Finchley, London, N2 9ED, United Kingdom
Str. Armeneasca 28/1, office 1, Chisinau MD-2012, Republic of Moldova, Europe
Printed at: see last page
ISBN: 978-620-7-91541-5

Contents

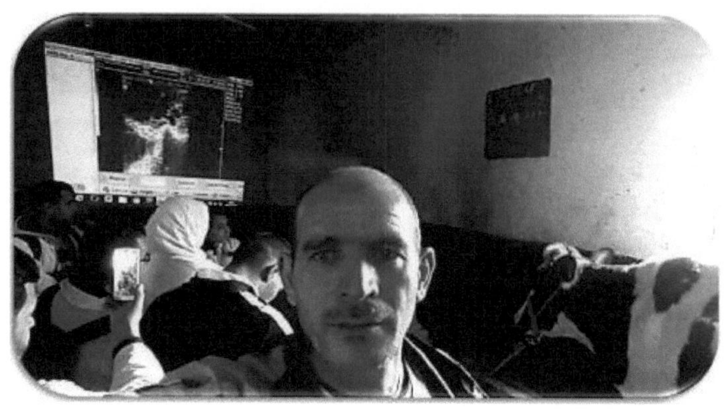

PREAMBLE

The "Reproductive pathology" module, which I describe as a "key module" in veterinary medicine, covers the most dominant and widespread pathologies in the various cattle farms, especially those intended for milk production.

This module deals with a very close relationship with reproduction, in addition to its role, interest and indispensable place in the socio-economic sector. It therefore occupies an extremely important place in bovine clinical practice in general, especially as nowadays the diseases and problems associated with the female bovine genitalia are increasingly accentuated and complex, requiring a good command of the subject for economic optimisation. This expertise, used in a special examination of the cow's genital tract, clearly helps us to understand the causes of these anomalies, known as aetiologies, and thus to establish a reliable and precise diagnosis. These precise diagnoses enable the best therapeutic methods to be chosen.

This manual is therefore aimed at veterinary students on the clinical cycle and practising veterinary surgeons working in rural clinics, mainly in the field of reproductive pathology in cows, who are looking to enhance their skills and

competencies in this area.
Doctor **ZEROUAL**. Fayçal

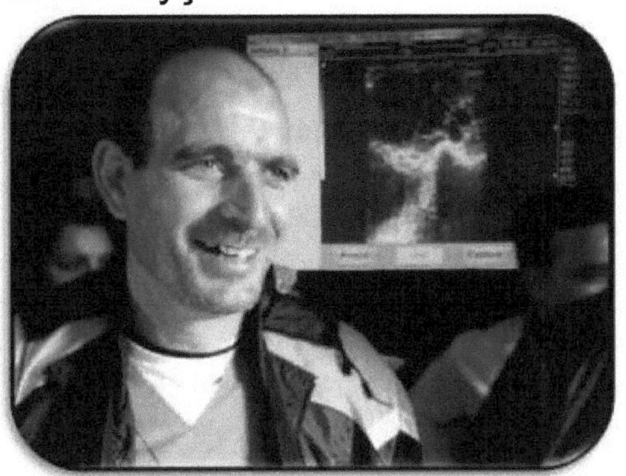

INTRODUCTION

The human lifestyle has evolved over hundreds of thousands of years from hunter-gatherer to farmer-breeder... This latter sedentary lifestyle therefore requires two things: mastery of production (animal and plant) in sufficient quantities (food) for an annual cycle and mastery of conservation and storage techniques for these same durations. Animal production, and more specifically cattle production, is constantly gaining in value and importance in veterinary medicine, particularly in terms of reproduction techniques. Self-sufficiency for society, mainly in red meat but also in milk, is a criterion for the development of agriculture, leading to the stabilisation of other socio-economic sectors in the country. From our point of view, achieving this self-sufficiency is closely linked to a good command and perfect knowledge of the veterinary field and reproductive pathology, as well as a mastery of farm management methods, since these are the cornerstone of successful breeding. Clinical examination of the female genital tract in cows is still one of the most difficult tasks for veterinary practitioners and students. It relies mainly on good scientific knowledge of the reproductive pathology module, as well as the correct use of certain specific tools and a better mastery of the rectal palpation technique, ultrasound exploration and para-clinics. This skill, which has become professional, is achieved through training and continuous and regular practical repetition, otherwise known as "professional experience". In fact, in order to achieve a good training and ensure a large harvest of knowledge allowing a better mastery of the act and the practice in this sense, we judged that the student in the clinical training sessions must first of all, manipulate on the real, that is to say before passing to the imaginary, which must be carried out using simple and easily assimilated methods, enabling them to successfully link and construct the reality of the images in such a way as to be able to distinguish between what is anatomo-physiological (normal) and what is anatomo-pathological (abnormal). To acquire and develop these technical gestures of rectal palpation, the clinician must carry out a large number of training sessions focusing on the basic landmarks of the genital tract, such as the vaginal cavity, cervix, body of the uterus, etc. In this case, the clinician or student must practise and carry out several clinical sessions on a maximum number of cow genitalia recovered from slaughterhouses from animals identified and screened ante-mortem. By the end of their training, these rehearsals will enable them to acquire a minimum of practical skills and knowledge that will enable them to make a definitive diagnosis.

1 CLINICAL EXAMINATION OF THE COW'S GENITAL TRACT

A/ Knowledge objectives

They aim to improve :

1. Mastery of a clinical examination of the female genital tract of a cow
2. Knowledge and exploration of the different anatomical parts of the genital tract
3. Diagnosis of pregnancy by rectal search
4. Making a probable diagnosis of a genital pathology
5. Making a differential diagnosis with other genital pathologies
6. Establishing a definite diagnosis
7. Choosing the right treatment for the disease

B/ Comprehension objectives

To have the right approach to take when faced with a clinical case in reproductive pathology, in order to establish a diagnosis of certainty that will enable the right therapeutic choice to be made and make the clinician's intervention as effective as possible.

C/ Application objectives

To know how to use and exploit the appropriate equipment and clinical means for female bovine genital exploration.

Successfully exploit and apply pre-acquired knowledge.

1.1 THE CLINICAL APPROACH

In addition to the theoretical knowledge acquired, good mastery of a clinical examination requires coordination and perfect use of the clinician's sense organs. Confirmation of the diagnoses made by veterinary clinicians is clearly the result of combining the right information on reproductive pathologies with the right stimulation of certain sense organs. For example, certain diseases such as metritis and acetonaemia can often be detected by the well-trained sense of smell (bad, foul, nauseating odour, etc.). On the other hand, vision, which plays a very important role here, can be used to distinguish abnormal tail carriage, discharge and genital secretions, as well as their nature and colour, which can only be seen with the naked eye. Vision can gather important information and observations such as oestrus, the nature of metritis, a sketch of the pelvis and the general condition of the animal. Present deformities and the overall condition of the vulva are additional information leading to the correct diagnosis. These findings certainly provide information on a number of pathological or physiological presentations, such as gestation, the case of a rear faix, uterine prolapse, vaginal prolapse, etc. Hearing in the examination of the female genital tract of the cow is of practically no interest because it is much more reserved for auscultation of the cardiopulmonary area and the digestive sphere. Sensation, otherwise known in the veterinary clinic as "palpation", can provide a great deal of information about the physiological and pathological state of the female genital tract. Examples include pregnancy, the functional or non-functional state of the ovaries, mummification, the presence or absence of cysts or corpus luteum, etc. Proper, well-organised conduct requires imperative compliance with all stages of the clinical examination, starting with the general before moving on to the special examination. Compliance with this approach generally leads to a good choice of treatment, based on confirmation of a definite diagnosis. It should be noted that, whatever the conditions, the cause, the obstacles or the arguments, the general clinical examination must be carried out at every consultation; under no circumstances should this absolutely necessary examination be neglected. It should also be remembered that good communication skills, whether with the breeder or the animal, greatly enhance the smooth running of our clinical examination. This communication, which has become a science of capital importance, must be introduced and even developed in veterinary medicine training programmes. The same applies to certain cases of psychological pathology, which are becoming just as important in veterinary medicine, such as pseudogestation in reproductive pathology.

1.2 CLINICAL EXAMINATION

1.2.1 Reason for consultation, history-taking and memorabilia

In reality, examination of the cow's female genital tract, like any other clinical examination, must begin with the first contact with the owner and the reason for consultation. This reason often determines the type and method of intervention chosen, and is used to better select and prepare the appropriate material for the clinical examination. During this initial contact, and throughout the operation, it is vital to avoid any confrontations that may arise between you and the owner, bearing in mind that a lack of communication, information, explanations, misinterpretations or even a refusal to declare the truth on the part of the breeder can have a negative impact on the smooth running of the clinical examination. For this reason, when you travel to the animal, it is preferable to bring as much equipment as possible that you consider essential at the time of the clinical examination of the female genital tract, since generally speaking several parameters such as time (availability of the clinician according to his programme), distance, degree of urgency and the state of the animal oblige you to be prepared and ready for any type of intervention. The clinician has to learn how to target his questions using simple, clear, understandable and uncomplicated language, so that messages can be passed on properly (avoid scientific terms and use terms that are familiar to breeders or breeders' vocabulary). At the same time, you need to gather as much information as possible, and above all, learn how to receive and filter information, co-ordinate messages received with your findings and acquired knowledge, and never deny, make the breeder lie or confront him (your mission is well defined: Combat, minimise suffering treat the animal). If the case arises or the veterinarian is monitoring a herd, it is well recommended to have a health monitoring form in paper or digital version, which permanently ensures the notification of all pathological events and includes all notes on the past reproductive life often called history of the animal (Dates of heat, artificial insemination, calving conditions, milk production ... etc.).

It should also be noted that anamnesis and memoranda make it possible to gather and collect as much information as possible about the animal's history or past, and to find out about any recurrences of pathological cases (dates and number of occurrences if necessary), interventions carried out by other vets, treatments undergone, vaccinations carried out, whether the animal has recently been introduced to the cowshed or not, the stages in the appearance of symptoms, syndromes and anomalies observed by the farmer, the animal's lifestyle, the feed ration (nature, composition, quantity and quality), etc.etc. Before starting a clinical examination, it is advisable to ascertain the animal's sex, although confusion between the two sexes in the bovine species is almost non-existent and is much more limited to certain pathologies such as free martinism and hermaphroditism. Age, on the other hand, can tell us a great deal about puberty, primi or pluri parturition. On the other hand, certain diseases are closely linked to the breed, such as white heifer disease (WHD), free martinism (twinning between male and female), the morphology of the animal and the pelvic girdle, which are much more closely linked to the cow's genetic potential (cases of dystocia), production (milk fever, ketosis) and its phenotype or morphotype (breed for milk or meat production).

1.3 GENERAL CLINICAL EXAMINATION

Mandatory and under no circumstances can it be eliminated or even neglected. It is always preferable to require the presence of the owner. The general clinical examination of the genital tract of the cow includes, in the majority of cases, the gynaecological examination and the obstetrical examination based essentially on an external and another internal examination, and is composed of :

1.3.1 External clinical examination :

It mainly starts with,

1.3.1.1 Remote inspection or remote clinical examination :

In fact, it is formally inadvisable to get close to an animal at the first attempt. An examination at a distance is a very fair and reasonable behaviour, which can clearly avoid many accidents, especially traumatic ones (defensive reactions of the animal for example) or incidents such as contractions of certain zoonotic diseases (Figures N°: 01 and 02).

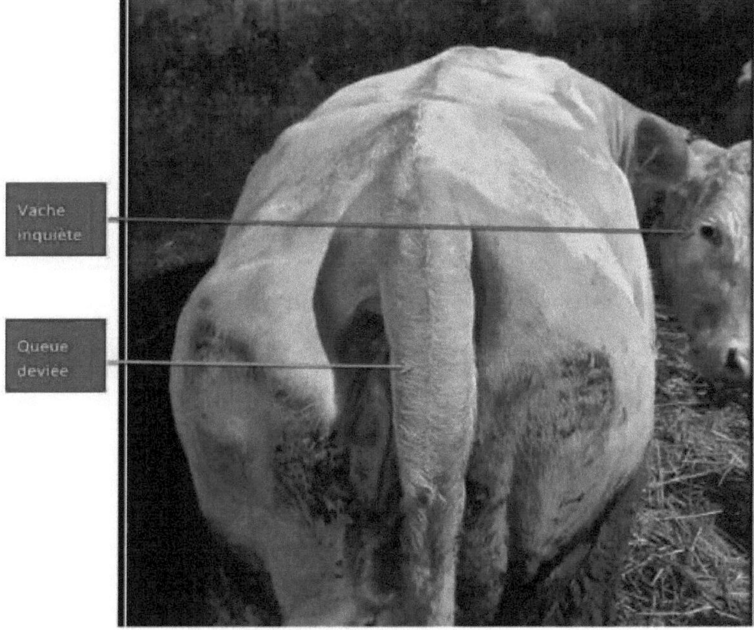

Figure 1: Remote inspection (Original photo 2016)

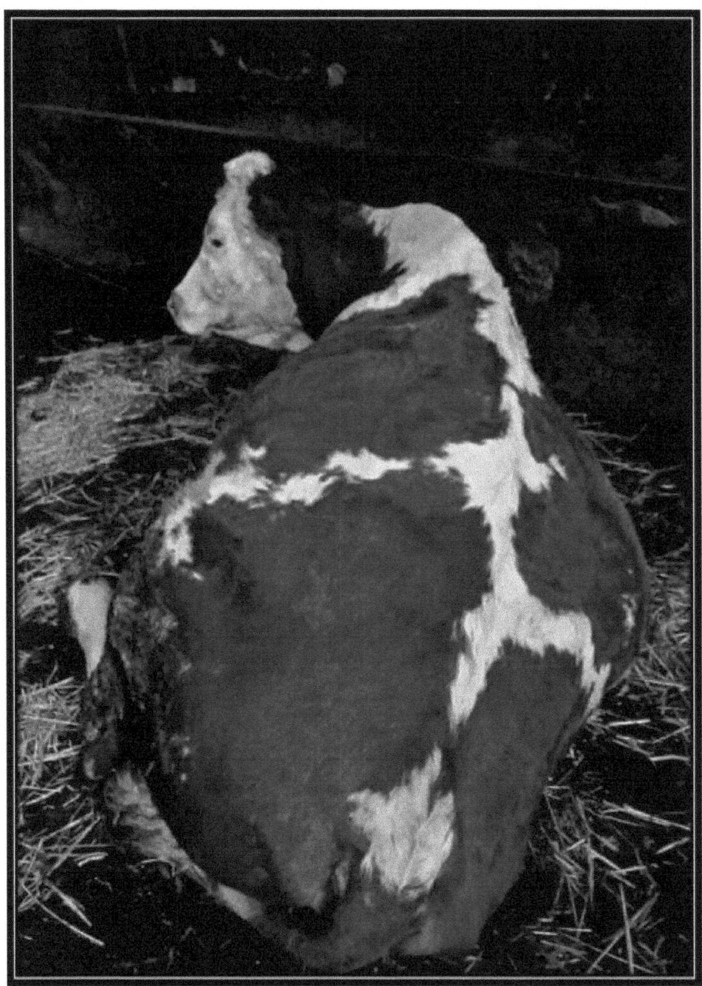

Figure 2. Cow in decubitus position (Original photo 2016)

On the other hand, work (examination) that is carried out gently and that takes into account all the measures of hygiene, safety, calm, luminosity, spacious, favourable and secure premises, clearly favours every kind of success (a good diagnosis or decision), gain (no contraction of zoonosis, no accidents and no incidents) and well-being (easy, simple and less tiring to carry out) for the clinician, the owner and the animal alike. It's best to start by inspecting the surroundings, the environment, checking for the presence or absence of foot baths and hygiene and prevention measures, whether or not the stable or place is well maintained, the situation, the presence or absence of neighbouring animals, the general state of the drinking troughs, feed troughs, feed ration (quantity and quality), aeration, cleaning, maintenance of the animals, state of the soil, irrigation, cultural level of the farmer, presence or absence of hygiene products (detergents and antiseptics).etc. Taking all these factors into consideration can provide extremely valuable information that is vital for clinical

examination; poor hygiene in fact clearly favours the appearance of vaginitis, metritis, cervicitis, salpingitis, mastitis, etc.).
During the clinical examination in reproductive pathology, inspection can provide us with information and help us to gather many of the key signs and symptoms needed to make a correct diagnosis. The animal presented at the gynaecology or obstetrics consultation is sad, in pain, apathetic, uninterested in its surroundings (unconscious), in an unusual position (self-auscultation, decubitus, spread hind legs, etc.). Wearing a smooth, dense and shiny coat (physiological), on the contrary, dull, broken, light, dishevelled, presence of depilation or alopecia (poor diet, mange, pediculosis, mycosis.etc). In a state of ecce or lack of stoutness (evaluation of the score, which can explain exposure for a long time to over- or under-feeding, parasitism, cachectising diseases (diarrhoea, tuberculosis, lameness, pneumonia or even hyper-milk production, etc.) (See Figure N°: 03).
Also check for the presence of deformities, any uterine hernia, damage to any anatomical region of the skeletal system which may indicate a fracture, separation or metabolic disease, etc., the presence of nodules (abscesses, cysts, haematomas, oedemas or even hypodermal larvae), or the presence of ectoparasites of the Ixodidae genus (ticks with assessment of the load of these haematophagous ectoparasites).

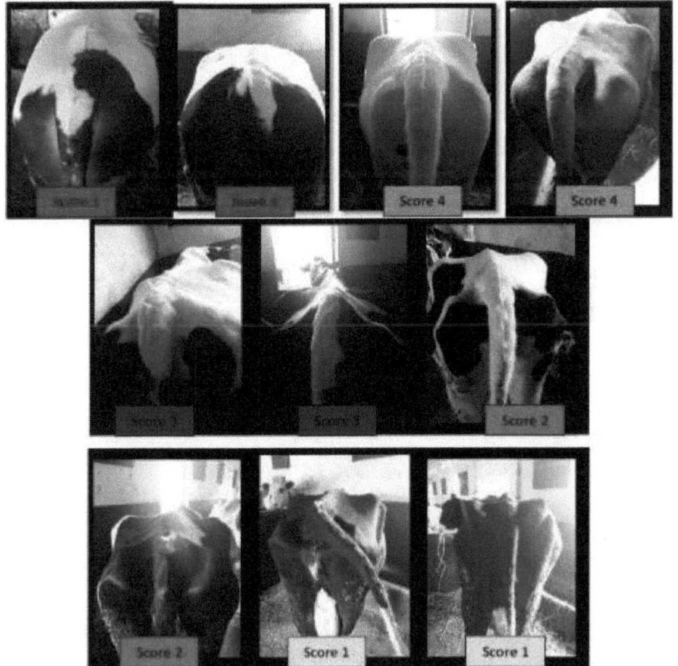

Figure 3. Overview of overweight cows from score 5 to score 1 (Original photo) 2016)

All these factors and others may indicate a consequence of malfunctioning in relation to the ovaries or immune deficiency, for example. The state of the labia may indicate oestrus or gestation (swollen and turgid), vulvitis or a bite (reptile, wasp, bee, etc.). A vulval discharge and, depending on its nature, whether or not the tail is raised and or deviated (see Figures 04 and 05) to the sides, which may indicate affections of the genital tract, or oestrus, or even gestation (denser colour).

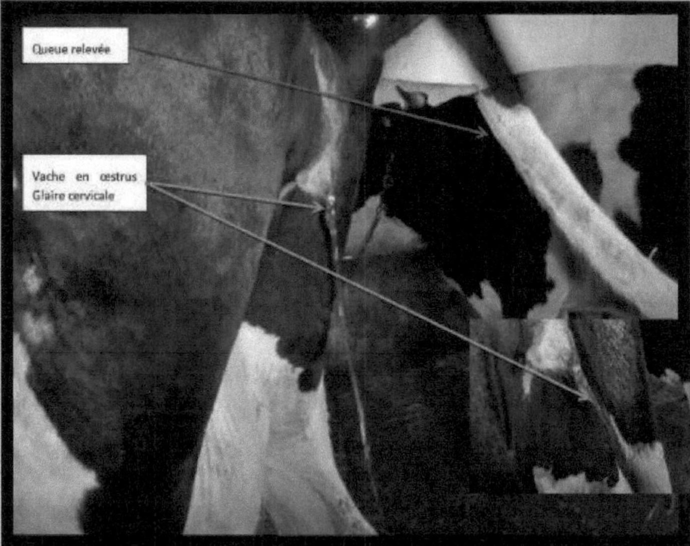

Figure 4. Cow in oestrus (Original photo 2015)

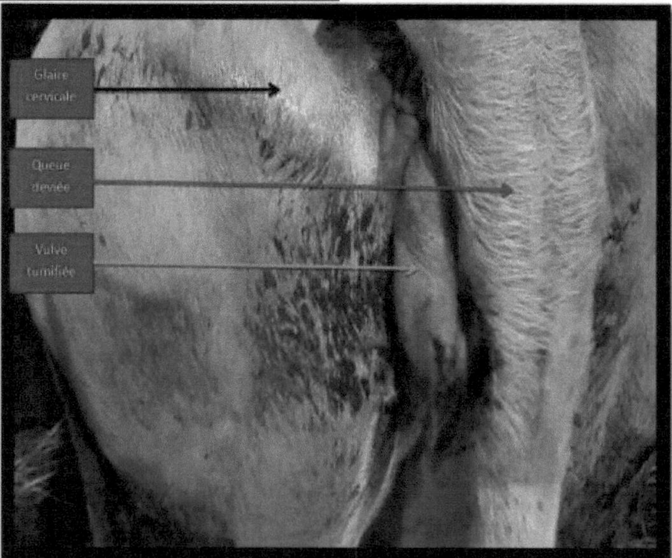

Figure 5. Swollen vulva (oestrus) (Original photo 2016)

Replenishment of the body, an arched back outside the usual urination, signals abdominal pain whatever its origin (animal crawling under itself) (See Figure 06).

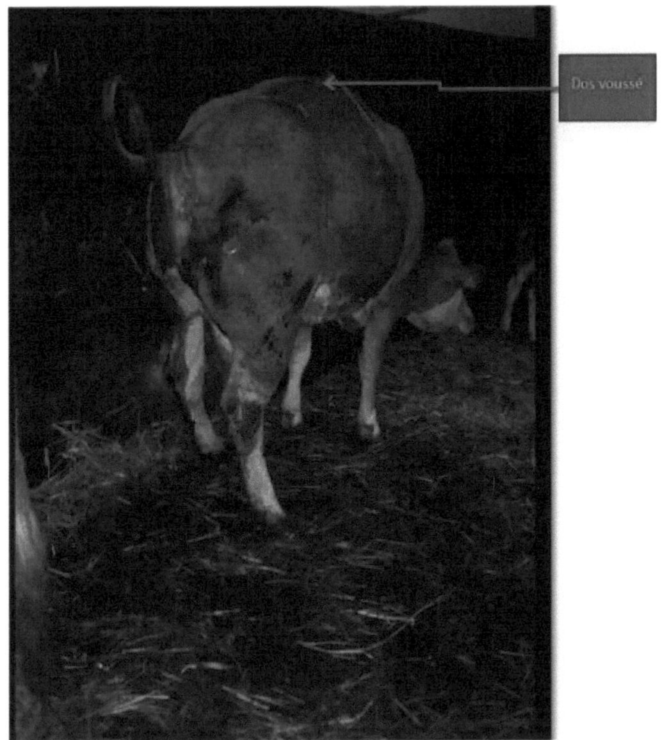

Figure 6. Arched back (Original photo 2016)

The clinician should inspect the symmetry of the pelvis (risk of deformities likely to interfere with parturition) and the state of the sacroischial ligaments. (See Figure 07).

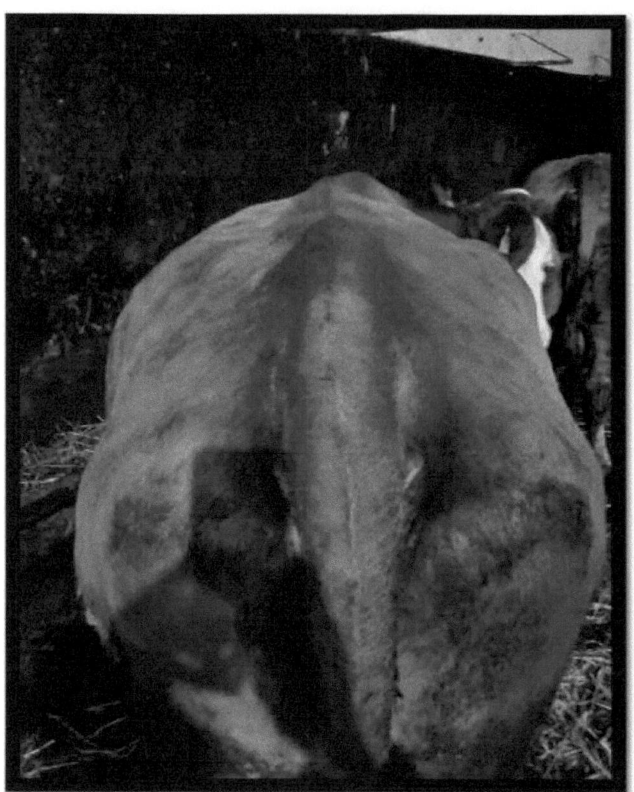

Figure 7. Overview of the symmetry of the basin (Original photo 2016)

Urination should be noted if it is normal or, on the contrary, difficult, and with pain, in addition to its nature as continuous micturition or drip by drip (oliguria), anuria, etc. These suggest above all damage to the urinary tract but can also sometimes be linked to a gynaecological problem (incomplete uterine involution, placental retention that is not visible, damage to the uterine mucosa, etc.) (Figure 08).

In the presence of agitation, continuous movements, trampling, consecutive lying down and rising, suggest imminent parturition or dystocia.

If you can't get up, don't rule out ante- or post-partum accidents, and think about pelvic fractures, sprains, muscle tears, ligament tendonitis, etc,

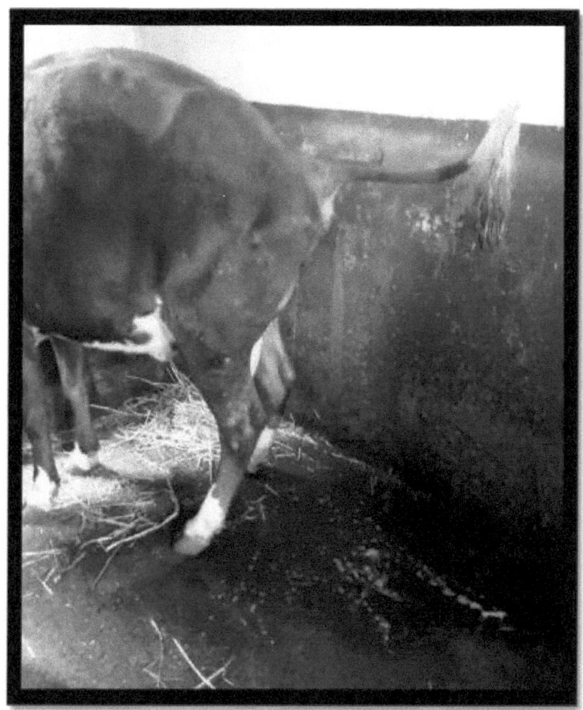

Figure 8. Urination (Original photo 2016)

In the event of vulval discharge or mucus discharge, note the colouration if it is white, viscous, translucent, sometimes located on a posterior part of the body at a maximum distance equal to the length of the tail or sometimes discarded on the ground which may indicate oestrus (Figure 09). This mucus can sometimes be denser and acrid white in colour, which may indicate gestation.

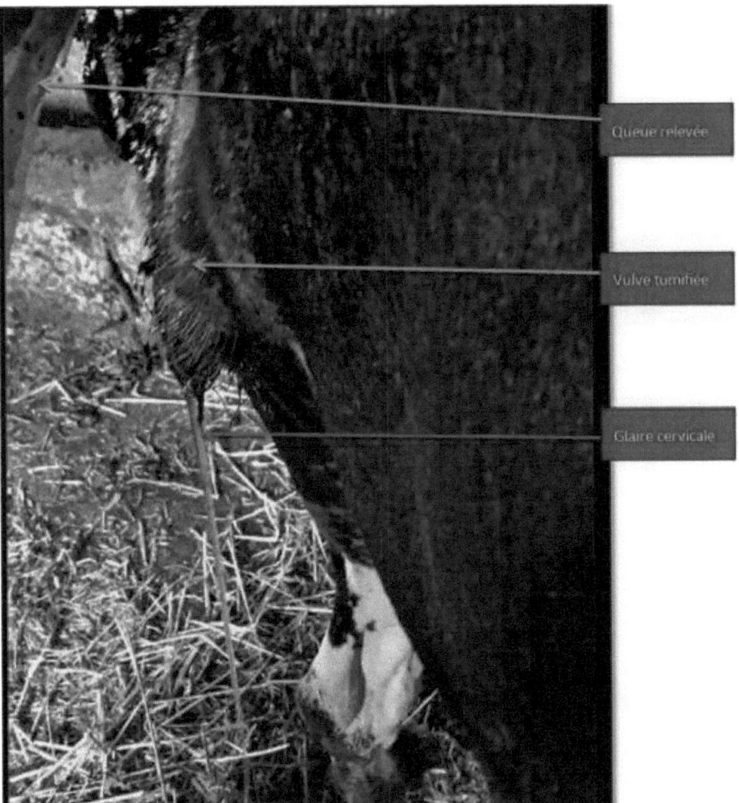

Figure 9. Cow in oestrus (Original photo 2015)

Other discharges may be detected: mucous, mucopurulent, purulent, fetid, putrefied or foul-smelling, in which case they indicate infectious damage to the genital tract (metritis, endometritis, maceration, rear faix, etc). Sometimes the discharge is bloody, indicating the end of heat, cotyledonary detachment or early abortion (Figures 10 and 11).

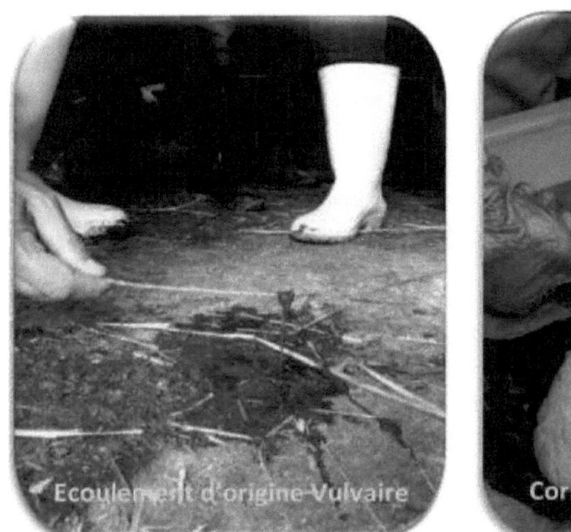

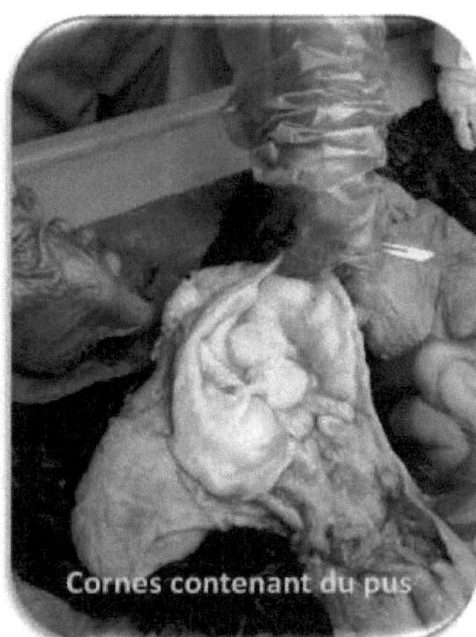

Figure 10. Different types of vulval discharge (Original photos 2016)

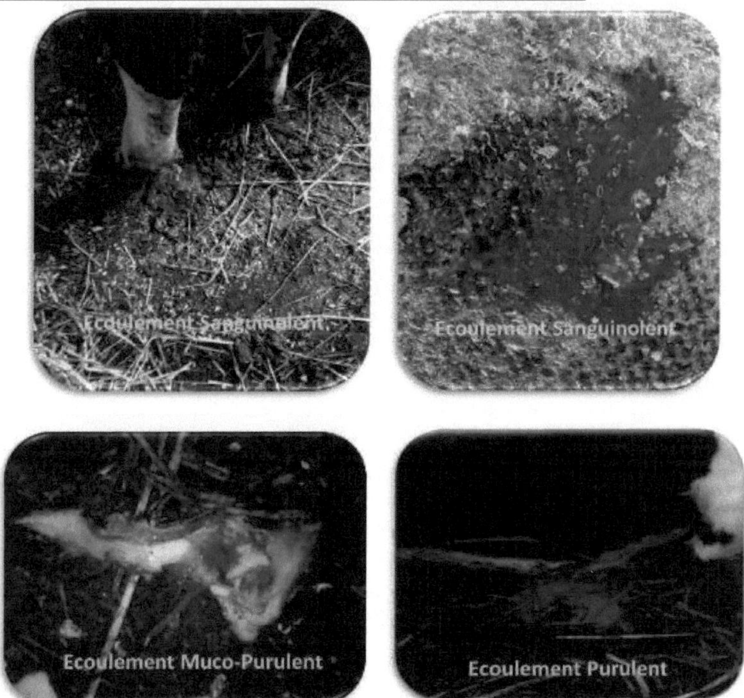

Figure 11. Different types of vulval discharge (Original photos 2015)

1.3.1.2 Close clinical examination :

In gynaecology, this examination is often referred to as a "close inspection".

A good inspection requires, above all, that the animal be properly restrained and that you keep your distance, because you should never approach a free animal, even if the owner insists that the animal is docile. Teach the breeder at least one method of derivative or physical restraint if he is not familiar with them. We can sometimes resort to chemical restraint if we deem it necessary (aggressive, dangerous, wild, very agitated animal, painful procedures, slow procedures, lack of help... etc).

Before approaching, it is advisable to take all the necessary safety and prevention measures (gloves, boots, preferably secure ones, etc.), to warn the animal by phonation (remind it of its name, for example, if it is named), to avoid sudden gestures and rapid movements (these can trigger reflexes or reactions in the animal that can be very dangerous), causing it to contract stress as well, etc. Leave a safe distance between you and the animal, be careful and take all kinds of precautions against possible kicks, headbutts, horns or trampling. These can cause accidents or leave serious after-effects. In general, it is preferable to start by approaching the animal from the front. On the contrary, if the animal is approached from behind, especially if it is poorly restrained, in most cases it will not let go and will seek confrontational positions from the front. Show the animal, a figure eight on the hocks is a good idea. Gently win the animal's trust by stroking it, even brushing it, to make it understand that you are not a source of danger or disturbance. Once the animal is well restrained, it undergoes the rest of the clinical examination: palpation, percussion and auscultation. Each examination proves its necessity and importance. Once these have been completed, we move on to the special clinical examination (gynaecological and/or obstetric). In general, depending on the case, a rectal palpation, an ultrasound scan or a vaginoscopy is performed.

Once close, lift the tail and examine the perineal area and the inside of the tail, looking for traces of secretions of genital origin (mucus or blood if perioestral or pus if pathological).

Palpate the anorectal lymph nodes on either side of the anus; if they are enlarged, they indicate local inflammation. The caudal edge of the sacro-ischial ligaments can be palpated between two fingers to check whether it is taut in normal cases, or relaxed a few hours before calving.

1.3.1.3 Inspection of the vulva

In the normal state, the vulva is generally vertical, and lies in the same plane as the tips of the ischium and the anus. It can sometimes be oblique when there is significant weight loss due to the melting of the fat pads of the perineum, because it follows the indentation of the anus, and in this case it seems to be "sucked" towards the abdomen. This oblique position can also be observed before calving due to the relaxation of the sacro-ischial ligaments, but becomes permanent and abnormal in certain multiparous females. The upper commissure of the vulva may disappear as a result of a tear following a dystocic parturition, in which case the anus and vulva are joined to form a cloaca.

Examination of the lower commissure reveals discharge from the genital tract: the hairs of the lower commissure are moist and stuck together by these secretions. Streaky, translucent discharge is a sign of oestrus, while more viscous mucus is seen when progesterone is present (particularly in diestrus). Brittle, cloudy or yellowish mucus is a sign of vaginal or uterine inflammation. It should be noted, however, that these discharges are often soiled by excrement and cannot always be interpreted. Inspection of the vulva also reveals the small clitoris. In free-martin cows, the labia of the vulva will be small, and the clitoris may be enlarged (Figure 12).

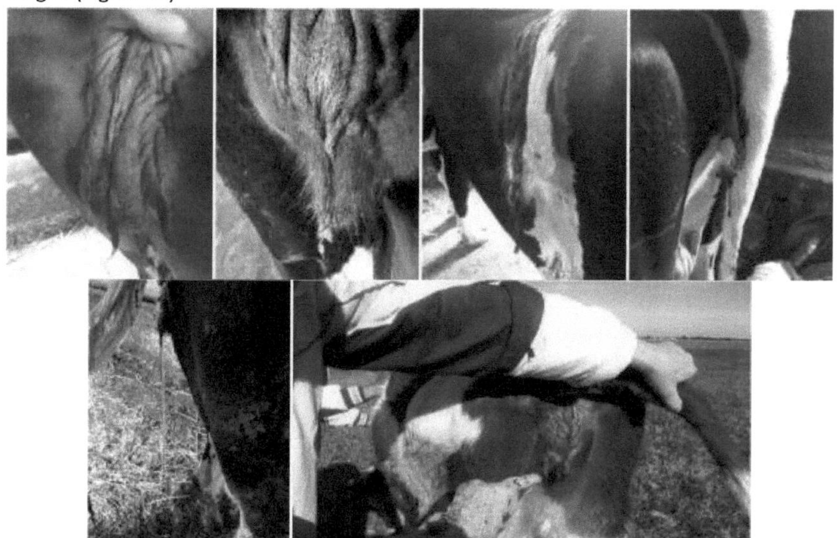

Figure 11: Inspection of the vulva (Original photos, 2012)

1.3.1.4 Internal inspection

The lips of the vulva, grasped between the thumb and forefinger, are spread apart, revealing the clitoris. This internal inspection enables the integrity and colouration of the vulvovestibular mucosa and the morphology of the clitoris to be assessed. The vestibular mucosa is normally pink, shiny and smooth. Hyperplasia of the lymphoid follicles gives the mucosa a bumpy appearance. These granulations may correspond to a normal inflammatory response of the vestibule to saprophytic flora, particularly in heifers, or to a reaction to specific pathogens (herpes virus, ureaplasma, etc.). This inspection can be carried out using a vaginoscope or a vaginal speculum accompanied by a light source, allowing examination of the vagina and the posterior part of the cervix, but its use can easily cause pneumovagina. In this case, never forget to clean the peri-genital area thoroughly, to avoid the onset of metritis or vaginitis. It is advisable to dip the speculum in an antiseptic solution, as its insertion may encounter vaginal bridles, persistent hymen or scarring stenoses that make it difficult to insert. The vagina may contain mucus (in heat), urine (urovagina), faeces (rectovaginal fistula) or pus (vaginitis or metritis). The posterior part of the cervix is rosette-shaped. In the luteal phase the cervix is firm and pale, in heat it is congested and open to about 1 to 2 cm in diameter, in which case it is called a "full bloom" (see Figure 13). Throughout gestation a mucous plug seals the cervix (see Figure 14), which softens and is expelled in the last week of gestation. Lochia (bloody secretions) can be observed 5 to 8 days after calving, and the same observation can be made after the cervix reopens for the first time 10 to 15 days later. It is also important to note that vaginoscopy can be used to monitor uterine involution, allowing early detection of endometritis, which can lead to failure to conceive and infertility.

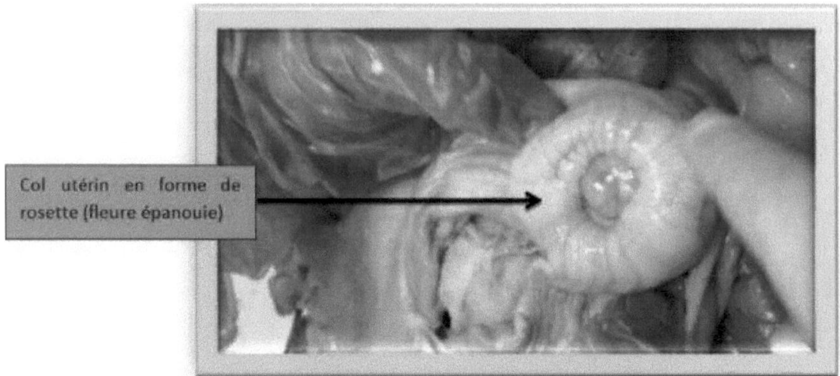

Figure 12. Uterine cervix (flower in full bloom) (Original photo, 2016)

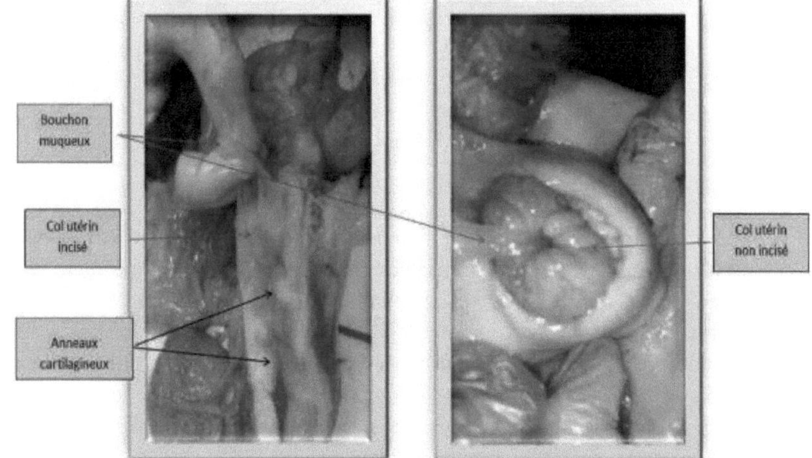

Figure 13. Mucous plug (Original photo 2016)

1.3.1.4.1 Palpation of the vulva

Vaginal palpation also requires the same hygiene precautions to be taken as vaginoscope insertion, but in this case it has the advantage of being quicker to perform than the previous procedure. The operator wears gloves that are soaked in clean water, which is used as a lubricant in this case. This allows any secretions to be collected. Palpation also reveals the thickness of the vulvar labia. The labia are small in free martin females (i.e. twins of a male) and in animals suffering from gonadal aplasia. On the other hand, they are more oedematous and flaccid in periods of heat or prepartum, and redder and thicker in cases of local inflammation.

The vulva can be subject to various deformations, tears, scars, following a difficult parting, abscesses or tumours (rare). These deformities can lead to poor lip contact, which can cause air to pass through when the animal is moved (pneumovagina). Vaginal exploration is also indicated during calving to check the opening of the cervix and the position of the calf, as well as the integrity of the cervix and vagina after birth.

1.3.1.4.2 Transrectal palpation

This propaedeutic method is one of the most important (Figures 15 and 16), since it can be used to :

- Examination of the genital tract,
- Diagnosis of pregnancy,
- Artificial insemination,
- Embryo harvesting and transfer,
- Intrauterine treatments,
- Tubal permeability test,
- Ultrasound-guided puncture,
- Obstetrical examination.

Before beginning the transrectal palpation operation, it is practically advisable to take all safety measures and precautions, to avoid any likelihood of contracting zoonoses, or other accidents or incidents.

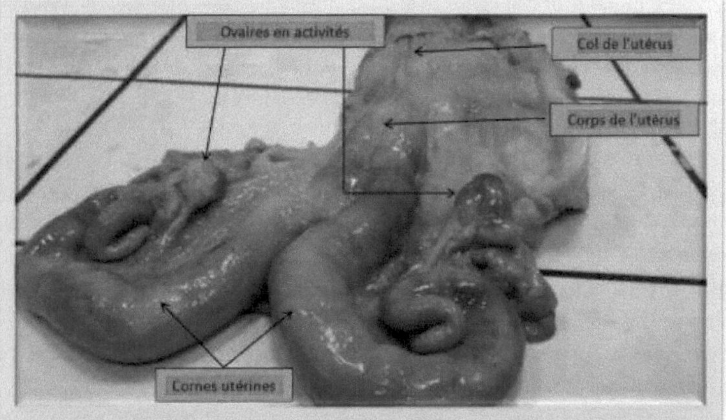

Figure 14. Female genitalia (cow) (Original photo 2016)

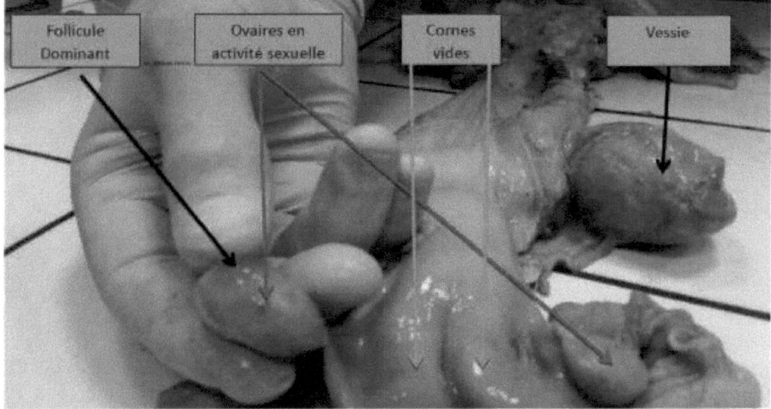

Figure 15. Empty female genitalia (cow) (Original photo 2016)

1.3.1.4.3 Palpation of the vagina

It is an odd, median, highly dilatable duct, with an average length of 30 cm and a width of no more than 5 to 6 cm in the cow. It extends forwards from the vestibule of the vagina and is inserted cranially around the uterine cervix, leaving a circular cul de sac around the cervix that varies in depth depending on the individual, known as the fornix of the vagina (absent in the sow but highly developed in the mare). The vaginal mucosa forms inconspicuous longitudinal folds, but above all radial folds forming a collar of three to five folds surrounding the vaginal opening of the cervix. Towards the rear, the vagina communicates with the vaginal vestibule via the ostium of the vagina, the perimeter of which is marked by a vestige of the hymen, a thin, incomplete partition of variable development more often distinct in mares and sows than in ruminants. The serosa only very partially covers the vagina in ruminants and sows (dorsal recto-vaginal cul-de-sac or cul-de-sac of Douglas and ventral vesico-vaginal cul-de-sac. In the mare, the cul-de-sac of Douglas covers the anterior third of the vagina. The muscularis is poorly developed. The mucosa comprises a stratified squamous epithelium. The number of cell layers increases during oestrus. Irrigation is provided by the vaginal artery. Sympathetic innervation is provided by the hypogastric nerve and parasympathetic innervation by the sacral nerves. Palpation of the vagina can identify pathologies such as pneumovagina, mucocolpos or tumours.

1.3.1.4.4 Palpation of the uterus

Commonly known as the womb (Metra), the uterus is the organ of gestation (see Figure 17). A hollow organ, it consists of two horns, a body and a neck. It is bipartitus in ruminants, with the two horns united caudally on a small portion or uterine body. On its own, the uterus weighs on average 400 grams (200 to 550 grams) and represents 1/1500th of the animal's live weight. The lining of the uterus is made up of three tunics, a serosa and a mucosa or endometrium. The endometrium comprises a simple epithelium and a propria. The thickness and oedema of the propria decrease during the progesterone phase of the cycle and increase during the oestrogen phase.

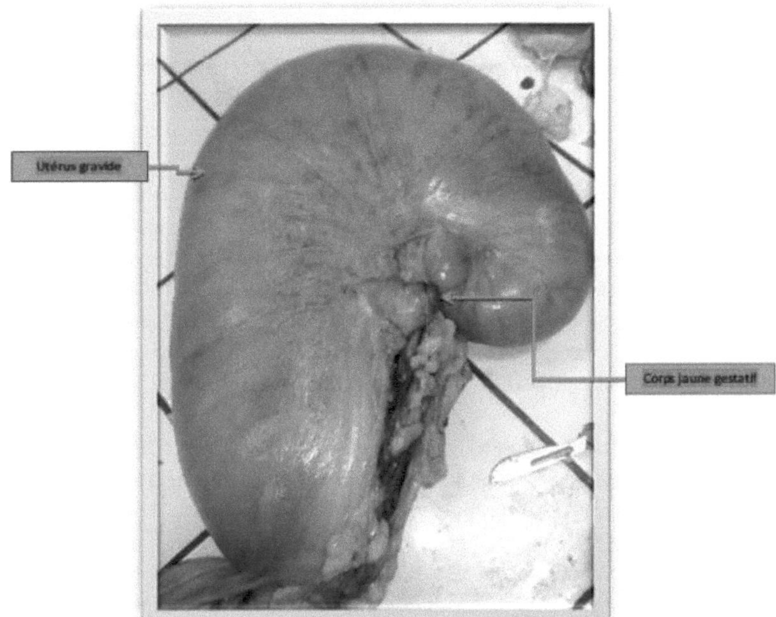

Figure 16. Pregnant uterus of a cow (Original photo 2016)

1.3.1.4.5 Palpation of the cervix

It is difficult to discern on the surface of an anatomical specimen. It is much longer (10 cm) than the uterine body. In cows, it is fibrous and has an internal structure known as a blossom, which makes it difficult to catheterise (pass through with a probe or insemination gun). The neck is shaped like a cylinder, 7 to 10 cm long, with a diameter of between 2 (heifer) and 5 cm (cow). The breed plays an important role in the variability of measurements. It can be more conical in shape, flaring out at the ectocervix. It is an essential reference point for the rest of the examination of the genital tract. Its position (pelvic, pubic or abdominal) and consistency (hard in the interoestral period, softening in the oestral period: differences in diameter (<5cm, 5-10cm or >10cm) are, however, barely perceptible) should be considered. Normally, the tip of the index finger should be able to touch the last joint of the thumb. It should usually be possible to mobilise the neck not only laterally but also anteroposteriorly. Retraction of the cervix not only allows any discharge from the vaginal cavity to be brought out, but also enables the presence or absence of abundant physiological (gestation of more than two months) or pathological (pyometra) fluids in the uterus to be assessed.

1.3.1.4.6 Palpation of the bifurcation of the horns

This is the best place to check whether or not the two uterine horns are symmetrical.

1.3.1.4.7 Palpation of the uterine horns

35 to 45 cm long in large cows (varying according to breed), the uterine horns gradually narrow towards the oviducts to which they join in the form of an S-shaped inflection. They have a diameter of 3 to 4 cm at their bases and 5 to 6 mm at their tips. Incurved in a spiral,

their apices are very divergent and located laterally more or less in the axis of the spiral. This positions the ovaries at the level of the cervix. Their mesometrial edge (small curvature) is concave and located ventrally in ruminants. Their free edge or large curvature is convex and located opposite the previous one. The two horns are joined at their base by two intercornuate ligaments, one ventral and the other dorsal, which is shorter than the first (Figure 18).

The uterus is mainly supplied by (1) the uterine artery, which originates at the beginning of the internal iliac artery, and (2) a uterine branch of the vaginal artery, which, like the internal pudendal artery, is derived more posteriorly from the internal iliac artery. The endometrium is reddish grey and usually has four longitudinal rows of caruncles, more prominent if the female has been pregnant, without glands, rounded or oval, slightly depressed in the centre in cows, whose volume increases considerably during gestation to form the foetal cotyledon. Palpation of the horns can also be used to diagnose gestation, but from 2[è] months for handlers with

experience, and later from 3[è] months for the less experienced (Figures 19, 20 and 21).

In addition to their presence (two or one: unicornuate uterus), it is important to check their consistency (flaccid, firm or tonic), mobility, diameter and position. The consistency of the horns is flaccid during the diestrous period. The horns are firmer in the proestrous period and during the first 72 hours of metestrus. They are toned in the oestrous period. In the cow, these changes in consistency are due more to changes in myometrial contractility. In the mare, on the other hand, the softening of the horns observed in the oestrous phase is due more to the oedematous state of the endometrium. The normal diameter of the horns is 2.5 cm (Surrounding the horn, the index finger joins the last joint of the thumb). It may be slightly larger (3.5 cm: surrounding the horn, the index finger reaches the tip of the thumb) in pluriparous women. Palpation of the horns along their greater curvature reveals adhesions, which in some cases appear as thicker or thinner and more or less extensive violin strings (flanges). It can also be used to identify the extent of healing of the internal caesarean section wound. The uterus can be manually retracted into the pelvic cavity in a number of ways: by grasping one or other of the uterine horns with the palm of the hand, with the fingers pointing backwards, trapping the uterus between the hand and the pelvis; by pulling on the intercornual ligament or the broad ligament. This retraction also has the advantage of facilitating the release of any physiological or pathological discharges.

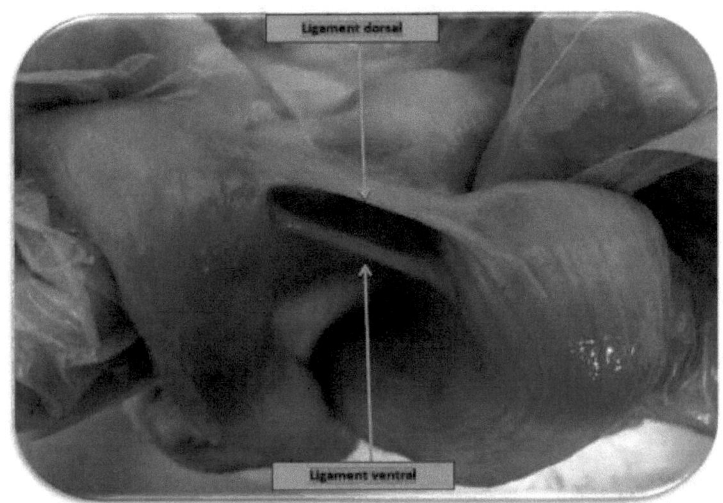

Figure 17. Intercornuate ligaments (Original photo 2016)

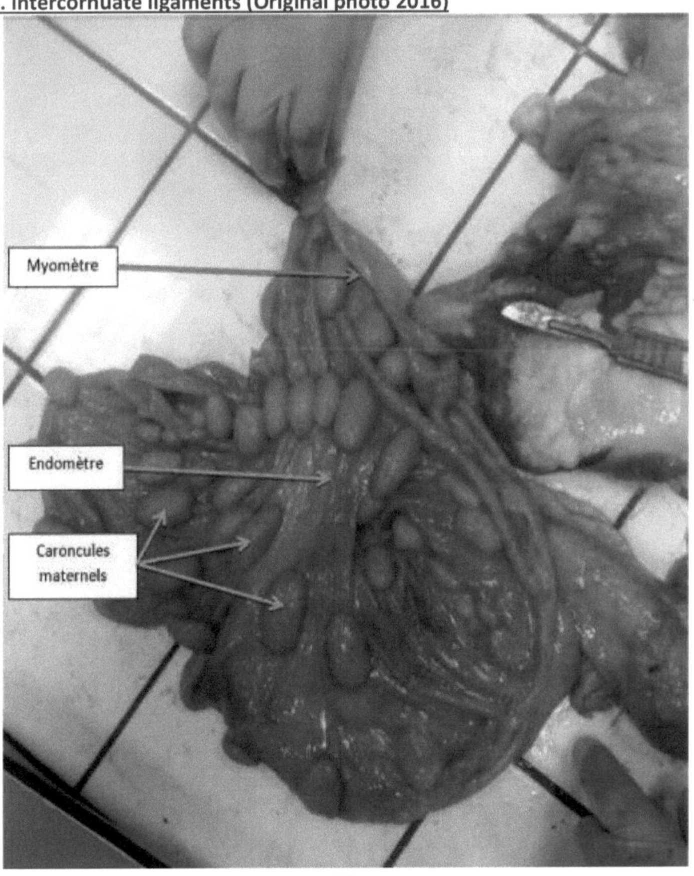

Figure 18. Pregnant female genitalia (cow) (Original photo 2016)

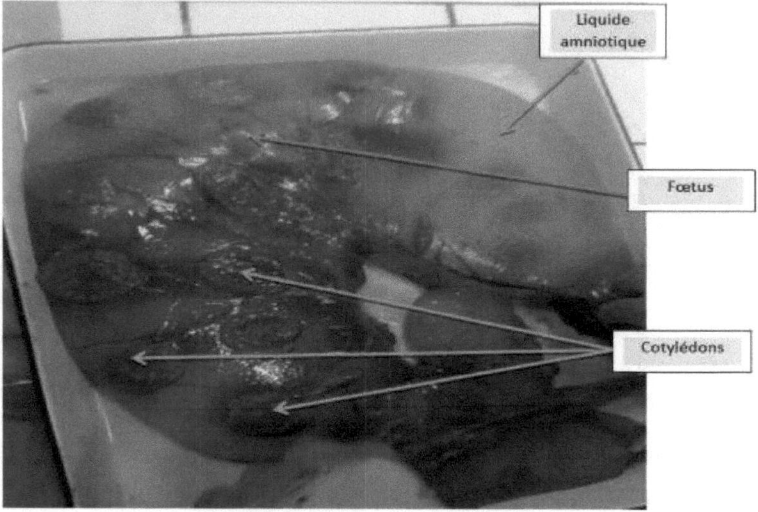

Figure 19. 05-month-old foetus (Cattle) (Original photo 2016)

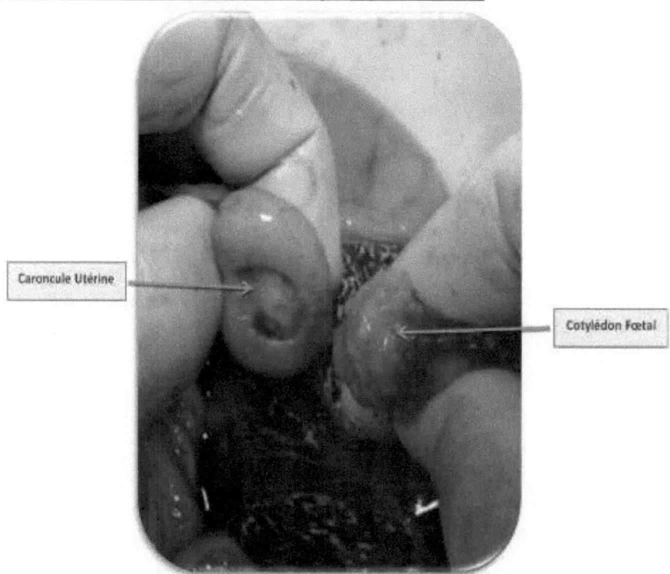

Figure 20. Placentome (Cattle) (Original photo 2016)

1.3.1.4.8 Palpation of the oviduct :

Also known as the uterine tube, salpinx or Fallopian tubes, it forms the initial part of the female genital tract. It receives the oocyte, where fertilisation and the first stages (D1 to D4 of gestation) of the embryo's development take place. The oviduct is very flexible, 30 cm long in cows and 3 to 4 mm in diameter. It is made up of an infundibulum opening onto the ovarian bursa, a clearly identifiable ampulla in the mare, and an isthmus 2 mm in diameter which gradually connects to the uterine horn. The oviduct comprises serosa, muscularis and mucosa. They are generally only palpable in pathological situations (salpingitis or cystic dilatation).

1.3.1.4.9 Palpation of the ovaries :

The size of the ovary varies according to the development of its functional structures. On average, it is 35 to 40 mm long, 20 to 25 mm high and 15 to 20 mm thick. It has a flattened, ovoid, almond-shaped form. It weighs 1 to 2 g at birth, 4 to 6 g at puberty and around 15 g in adults (10 to 20 g). In general, the right ovary is 2 to 3 g heavier than the left.
The ovary has a free rim and a rim to which the mesovarium is attached. This area of the hilum is vascularised extensively and should not be confused with the ovarian follicles during ultrasound examination. The ovary has a central vascular zone (medulla) and a peripheral parenchymal zone (cortex).
The ovarian bursa is delimited by the mesovarium, which suspends the ovary, and by the mesosalpinx, which fixes the oviduct close to the ovary. The ovary is irrigated by the ovarian artery, which arises from the caudal part of the abdominal aorta. Before reaching the ovary, it delegates a small uterine branch. After numerous branches, it reaches the hilum of the ovary through the mesovarium. The uterine vein coexists closely with the ovarian artery. This plexus is directly involved in regulating the cycle, with prostaglandin F2alpha passing in the cow directly from the uterine vein into the ovarian artery. The ovary contains several types of physiological organelles: follicles and corpora lutea. In both cases, there are several types, each with its own anatomical and hormonal characteristics. These structures coexist throughout the cycle and interact to regulate it. They are usually located approximately one handbreadth in front of and to the side of the anterior end of the cervix. They are usually grasped between the index and middle fingers so that they can be palpated with the thumb. The ovaries are most often identified by following the horns to their tip. As a general rule, the ovaries are clearly distinguishable from the ovarian bursa. If this is not the case, the reason may be the presence of PID. The first step is to assess the consistency (smooth or granular) and size (small: 0.5 cm or normal: 2 to 3 cm) of the ovaries. Granular consistency indicates a certain level of ovarian activity, i.e. the presence of primary, secondary or even tertiary follicles. Asymmetry of the ovaries should suggest the presence of a normal functional structure (De Graaf follicle, corpus luteum) or pathological structure (cysts) on the larger ovary. Secondly, we look for the presence of physiological or pathological structures. It should be remembered that the history, palpation of the uterus and vaginal examination are important aids in interpreting the ovarian structures found.

- Follicles are classified as primordial (0.04 mm), primary (0.06 to 0.12 mm), secondary (0.12 to 0.2 mm), tertiary (0.3 to 2 mm), pre-ovulatory (2 to 20 mm) and De Graaf (20 to 25 mm). Histologically, only the pre-ovulatory and De Graaf follicles are cavitary and therefore visible by ultrasound. Anatomically, only the pre-ovulatory and De Graaf follicles can be palpated manually.
- The mature follicle is about 2 cm in size and should not exceed 2.5 cm; once this size is exceeded it is known as a follicular cyst. It is therefore smooth and fluctuating. Its depressive nature is accentuated during oestrus. It is accompanied by a tonic state of the uterus (see Figure 22). Immature follicles are present at all stages of the cycle or gestation. They may coexist with a functional corpus luteum, but in this case the uterus is not tonic. Only follicles

larger than 1 cm can be truly diagnosed. The number of follicles larger than 1 cm in diameter is particularly increased after superovulation treatment.

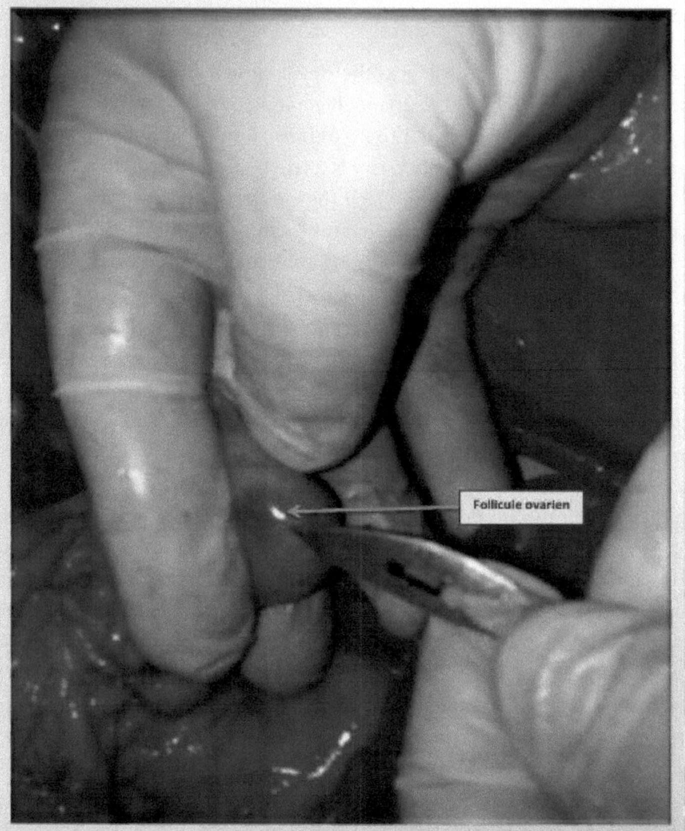

Figure 21. Ovarian follicle (Cattle) (Original photo 2016)

- During ovulation, the follicle decreases in volume, its wall wrinkles and its cavity fills with a sero-fibrinous exudate which soon coagulates. This is followed by major capillary neoformation on the one hand and major multiplication and transformation of the granular cells into luteal cells (luteocytes) on the other. During this phase of development (the first days of metestrus), the initial coagulum becomes infiltrated with blood, justifying the name haemorrhagic corpus luteum or red body given to this dark red or even blackish structure. Two types of cells gradually multiply, some derived from the granulosa (large luteal cells) and others from the theca (small luteal cells). After a few days, these cells push all or part of the coagulum back towards the centre, where it persists in the form of a simple trail or in the form of a cavity or smaller cavity such as that seen in cavitary corpora lutea. The luteal cells are simultaneously charged with a carotenoid pigment, lutein, which gives the fully developed corpus luteum its characteristic orange or even yellow hue. This pigment is more brownish in small ruminants and sows. The corpus luteum then reaches a size of 20 to 25 mm wide and 25 to 30 or even 35 mm long. Towards the end of diestrus, the corpus luteum gradually recedes. It takes on a more rusty hue, its surface protrusion (stigma) is gradually reduced, and it undergoes fibrous then fibrohyaline degeneration, giving it a whitish appearance (corpus albicans).

The corpus luteum as such, i.e. present during the diestrous phase of the cycle, is only really palpable between the 6th and 18th day following oestrus or during gestation. Its consistency is similar to that of a normal liver. It is 2 to 3 cm in diameter (see Figure 23). It may protrude from the surface of the ovary and thus stand out more or less clearly depending on the case. Their number may be increased after superovulation treatment. From the 3rd or 4th day of the cycle, it is already possible to detect a slightly protruding structure on the surface of the ovary, more or less small (< 2 cm) and soft: this is the haemorrhagic corpus luteum. It is also possible to palpate hard structures the size of a pinhead, called corpus albicans, corresponding to former involuted and therefore non-functional corpus luteum. Finally, by ultrasound examination it is possible to identify the presence within the corpus luteum of a cavity of varying diameter, which justifies the name of cavitary corpus luteum given to these structures. (See figure N°24). It is possible to enucleate the corpus luteum by palpation. This practice has been abandoned since the advent of prostaglandins. It is not without risk of haemorrhage.

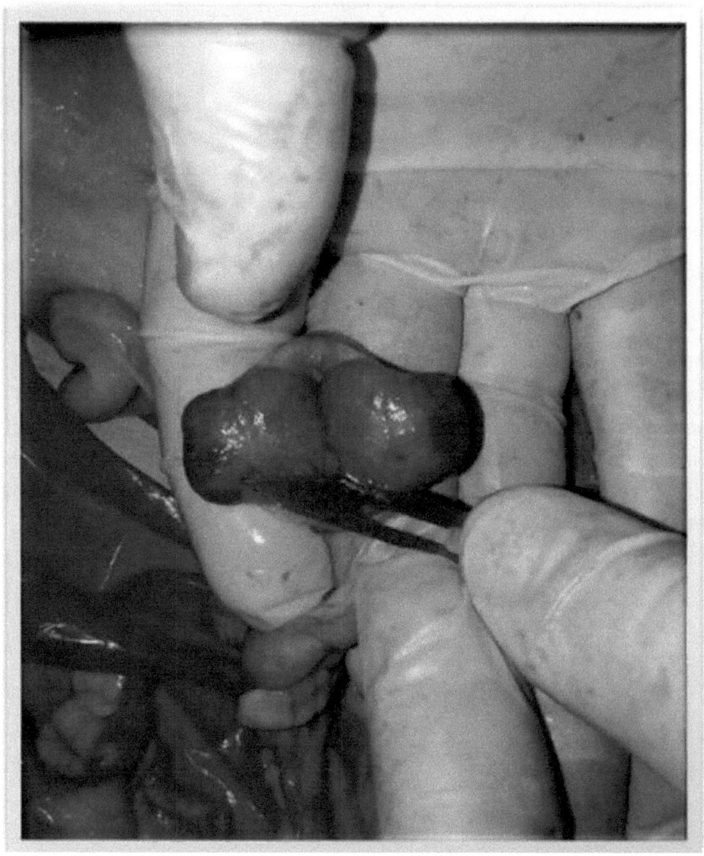

Figure 22. Yellow body (Cattle) (Original photo 2016)

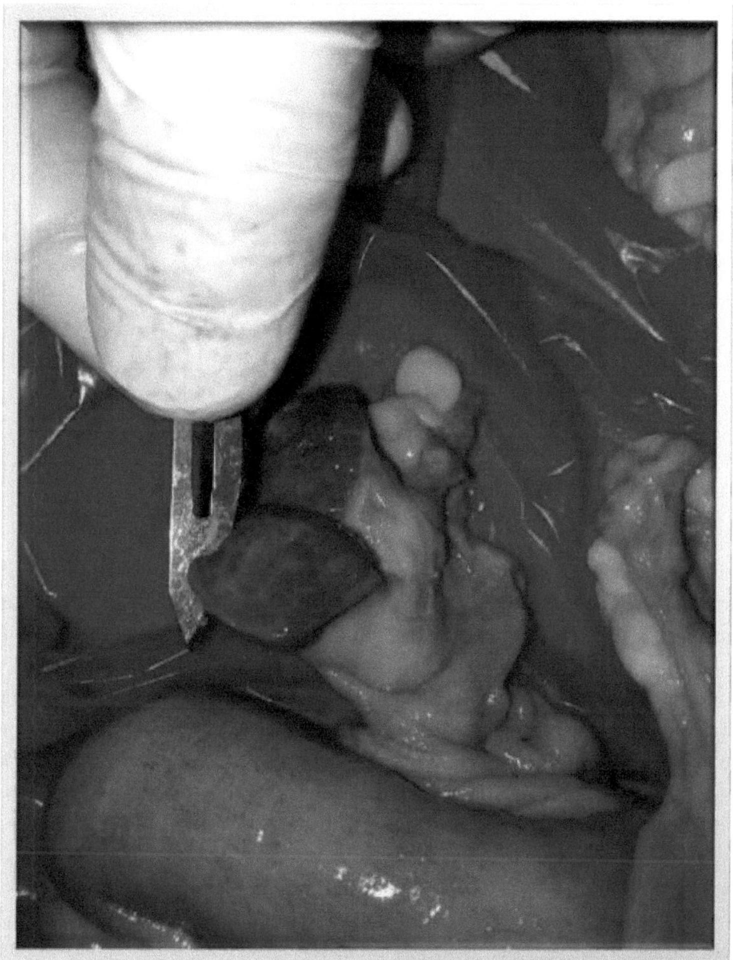

Figure 23. Cavity corpus luteum (Cattle) (Original photo 2016)

- The follicular cyst or cystic follicle (see figure 25) has the same characteristics as the mature follicle. However, in most cases it is larger than 2.5 cm. It is more resistant to pressure.
- Diagnosis of the luteinised cystic follicle or luteal cyst is much more difficult. It feels more fluctuating than the corpus luteum. It is also generally larger in size.

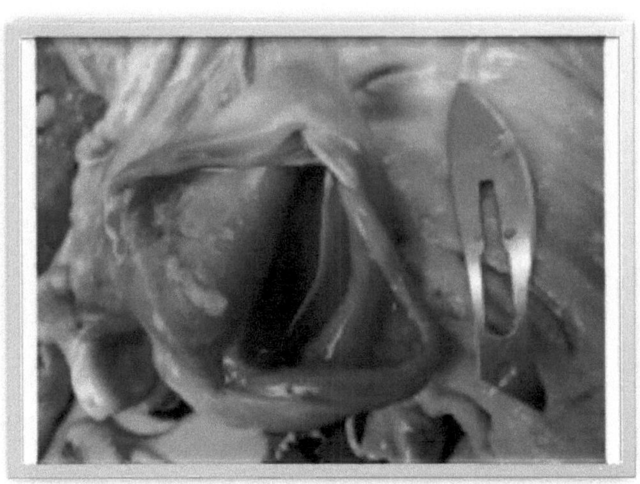

Figure 24. Incised luteinised follicular cyst (Hanzen 2015)

1.4 ULTRASOUND

Ultrasound is a reliable, non-invasive technique that is an invaluable tool for monitoring the oestrous cycle and diagnosing genital pathologies in cows. This technique is used routinely in veterinary medicine, but requires the practising veterinarian to be proficient both in performing the ultrasound scan and in interpreting the images.

It uses ultrasound waves to produce images. Ultrasound is a mechanical vibration of the same nature as sound waves, but with a higher frequency. In veterinary medicine, the range of frequencies used is between 3.5 and 10 MHz. The ultrasound intensity used is low and therefore harmless to the animal. The speed of propagation of ultrasound waves depends on the medium in question: it increases with the molecular cohesion of the tissue passed through. Descartes' laws concerning the reflection and refraction of light waves at a dioptre are directly applicable to ultrasound waves. Ultrasound is produced by the piezoelectric crystals of the probe, which vibrate under the effect of an alternating electric current, thus creating an acoustic signal, i.e. a deformation of the underlying molecules. The ultrasound waves are emitted in bursts over a very short period of time and propagate through the area to be scanned. Reflection, which is the basis of the ultrasound image, occurs when the wave encounters an interface between two media with different acoustic impedances. Acoustic impedance reflects the ability of a medium to propagate ultrasound, which corresponds to the product of the speed of the wave and the density of the medium. At the interface between two media with different acoustic impedances, part of the wave's energy is reflected and forms an echo, while the other part is transmitted across the interface and can explore the underlying tissue (see Figure 26).

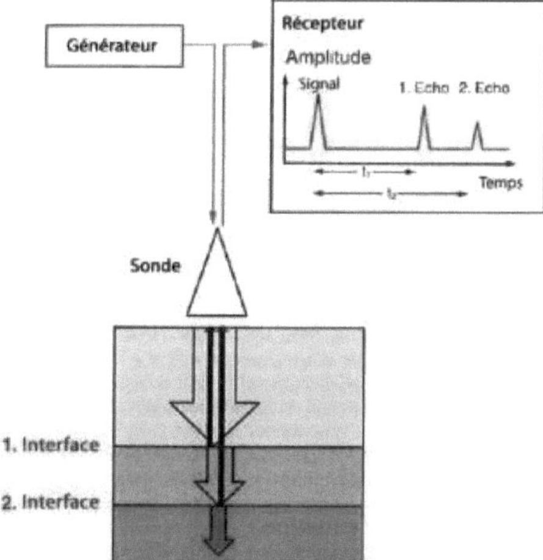

Figure 25. Principle of echo formation (Barr, 2011)

The greater the difference in impedance between two media, the greater the intensity of the echo, as in the case of a bone-tissue interface, for example. When reflected, the echoes produced return to the piezoelectric crystals, which vibrate and generate an electrical signal. A crystal is therefore both a transmitter and receiver of ultrasound waves. The delay between the propagation of the ultrasound and the reception of its echo determines the distance between the probe and the interface.

The ultrasound produced by the vibrations of the piezoelectric crystal is reflected by an acoustic interface, i.e. an interface between two media with different acoustic impedances. The reflected wave or echo returns to the piezoelectric crystal and generates a current in response to the reception of the echo. The delay between the propagation of the ultrasound and the reception of its echo is used to determine the distance between the crystals and the interface. The energy of the wave is attenuated as it propagates through the tissue, so the intensity of the echoes decreases with depth.

Ultrasound passing through homogeneous liquids (urine, amniotic and allantoic fluid, follicular fluid, blood) does not encounter any interfaces, and these areas will give anechoic, black or very dark images. On the other hand, in liquids containing particles in suspension (such as pus), ultrasound will encounter multiple small interfaces, which will form small echogenic and mobile spots on the screen, the result of the diffraction phenomenon.

Soft tissues (the uterus, for example) constitute echogenic zones represented by shades of grey according to their density: ultrasound undergoes so-called specular and non-specular reflections.

- A specular reflection occurs when the beam falls on a smooth surface that is wider than the beam and parallel to the probe. In this case, the amplitude of the echo depends not only on the difference in acoustic impedance, but also on the angle of impact. This is the case, for example, of the folds in the wall of the cervix (ultrasound image 1) and the surface of ovarian follicles.
- Non-specular reflections are caused by reflections from surfaces that are rough or narrower than the beam. In this case, the amplitude of the echo does not depend on the

angle of incidence of the beam. Parenchymal structures, particularly the corpus luteum, are the source of non-specular echoes, so the corpus luteum appears as a homogeneous grey structure, with a relatively constant shade of grey whatever the orientation of the probe.

Bone and cartilage reflect almost all ultrasound: they therefore act as obstacles to ultrasound, and appear as hyperechoic structures on the screen.

1.4.1 ULTRASOUND IN THE GENITAL TRACT OF THE COW

Ultrasound is a diagnostic tool commonly used by practising veterinary surgeons, particularly when monitoring reproduction on cattle farms. It can be used to accurately diagnose various physiological situations (ovarian monitoring and gestation) or pathological situations in bovine gynaecology.

Ultrasonography of the cow's reproductive tract is a valuable aid in the management of reproduction and the diagnosis of pathologies of the cow's reproductive tract. The aim of this section is to guide the operator in the interpretation of ultrasound images by presenting the current possibilities of application in bovine gynaecology, through images of the genital tract during different physiological and pathological situations. (See figure 27).

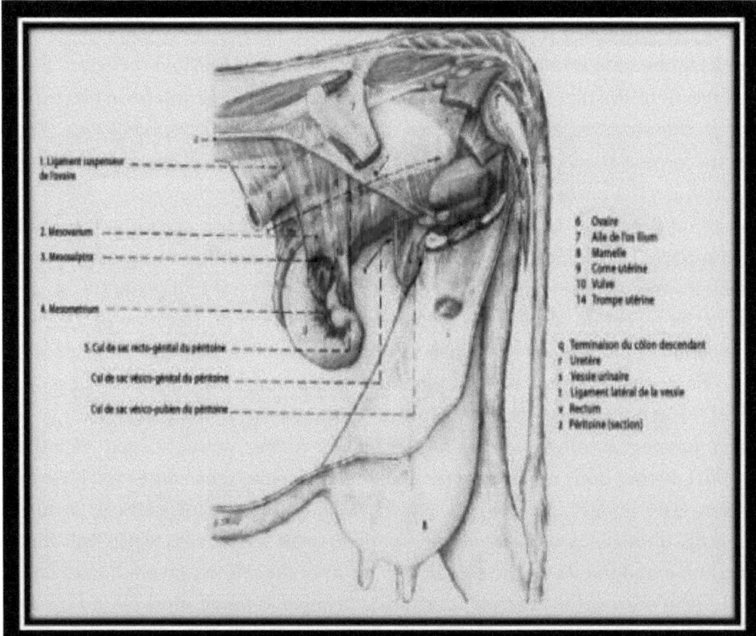

<u>Figure 26. Anatomy of the cow's genital tract (Burdas 2003)</u>

1.4.1.1 Ultrasound examination of the non-pregnant genital tract

Ultrasound of the bovine genital tract is performed transrectally. This examination technique is inseparable from transrectal palpation. Various anatomical landmarks help to orientate the probe as it progresses through the rectum. After passing through the anus, the bladder is visualised as a hollow organ filled with anechoic fluid, either oblong or circular in shape. Beneath the bladder, the bony components of the pelvis appear as an echogenic structure a few millimetres thick. The cervix is then identified by the circular folds and the cervical canal, which is 7 to 10 cm long and shows a strong horizontal linear echo. Moving cranially, the uterus is accessed. To ultrasound the ovaries, the ultrasound probe is placed at the level of the bifurcation of the uterine horns and then deflected in its longitudinal axis, laterally towards the ascending branch of the ilium. The ovaries are generally visualised in this direction. However, ovaries in cows are relatively mobile and are not always visible at the angle of the probe. In this case, the technique involves holding the probe in the palm of the hand to be palpated and grasping the ovary with the fingertips. The ovary will then be pressed against the ascending branch of the ilium and the ultrasound probe placed over it.

1.4.1.2 The genital tract during the oestrous cycle

1.4.1.2.1 The ovaries

The ovaries are generally located ventrally to the iliac bone, at the bifurcation of the horns. The ovary is almond-shaped, around 3 to 5 cm long and 2 to 2.5 cm thick. It contains peripheral organelles (follicles and corpus luteum) within the ovarian stroma. The medulla has a homogenous ultrasound appearance, whereas the ovarian cortex is heterogeneous due to the presence of ovarian organelles or blood vessels. With ultrasound equipment of average resolution, it is sometimes difficult to distinguish the outline of the ovary from the adjacent soft tissue. (See Figure 28).

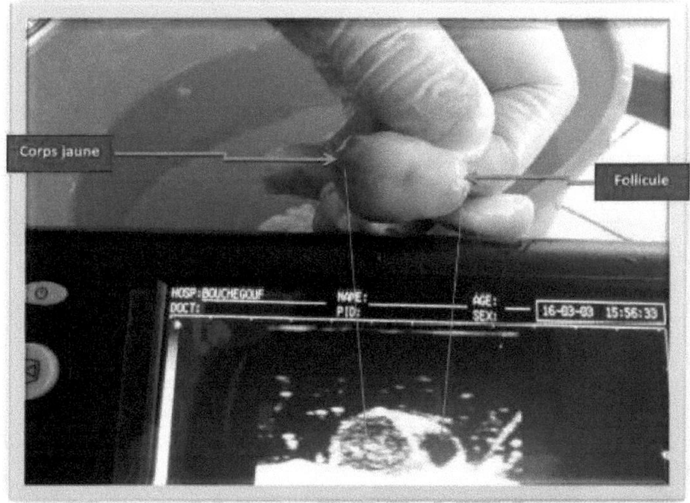

Figure 27. Image of ovary on ultrasound (Original photo 2016)

1.4.1.3 Presentation of the different ovarian organelles

1.4.1.3.1 Follicles

The follicles appear as spherical vesicles with a fluid content, thin-walled and flush with the surface of the ovary. On ultrasound, the follicle appears anechoic, in the form of a round area (or slightly elliptical under the pressure of the probe, or due to contact with an adjacent follicle). On an ovary, it is possible to identify one or more follicles, which vary in size depending on their stage of growth. Their diameter varies from 3 mm (minimum size of the follicle easily identifiable on ultrasound with a 10 MHz probe, given the power of resolution), up to 20 mm (for the pre-ovulatory follicle) with a maximum of 25 mm, once this measurement is exceeded we are faced with a case of follicular cyst. (See figures 29, 30 and

31).

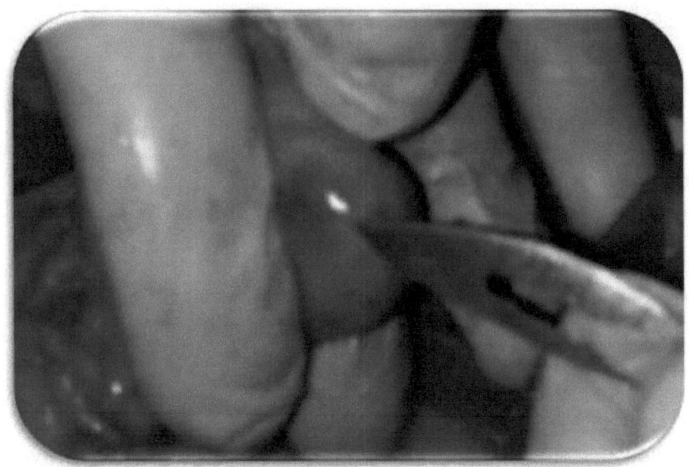

Figure 28. Ovarian follicle (Original photo 2016)

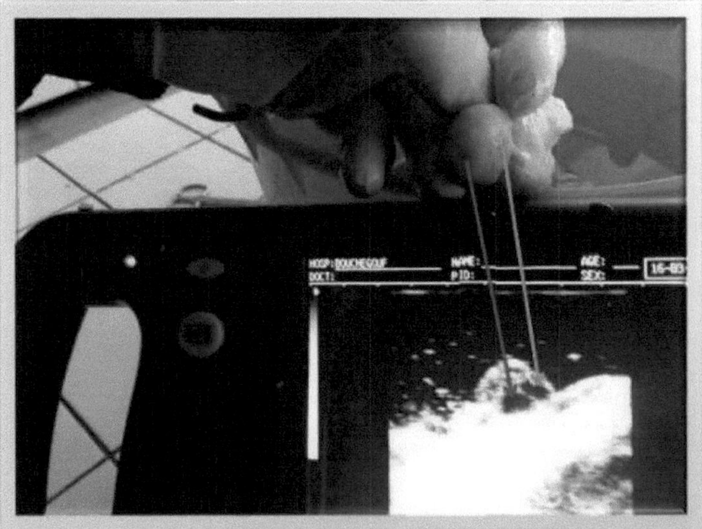

Figure 30: Ultrasound image of ovary with follicles (Original photo 2016)

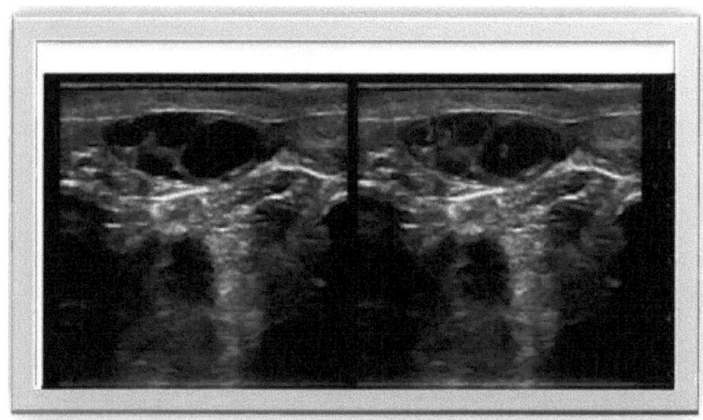

Figure 29. ultrasound image of ovary showing 5 follicles of different sizes

1: Ovarian stroma - 2: Follicles of different sizes (Scale: one scale corresponds to 0.5 cm) (Taveau and Julia 2013)

The differential diagnosis must be made with a follicular cyst (see Figures 32, 33 and 34), which is larger than 25 mm. It is also important to distinguish between a follicle and a cross-section of a blood vessel: by changing the orientation of the probe so as to obtain a longitudinal section, the image of the vessel will stretch, whereas that of the follicle will remain spherical and gradually diminish.

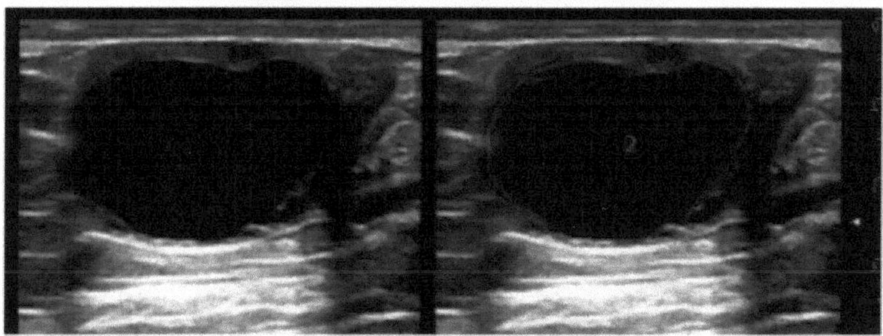

Figure 30. Ultrasound image of ovary with follicular cyst. Scale: one scale corresponds to 0.5 cm.

(Taveau and Julia 2013)

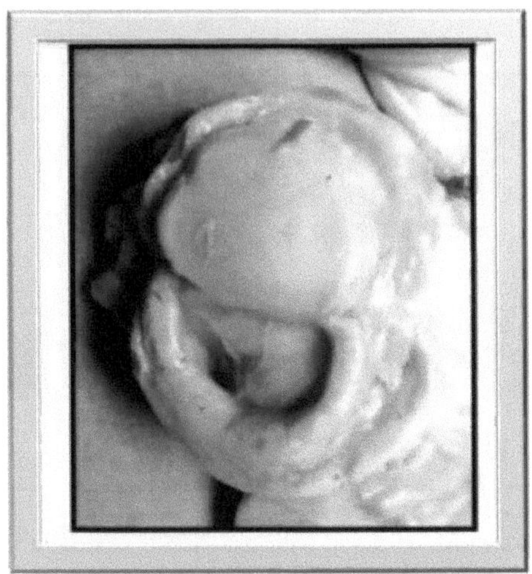

Figure 31. Luteal cyst. Wall > 3 mm (Reproduction unit, ENVA)

[Dornier P and Droui X (2013)]

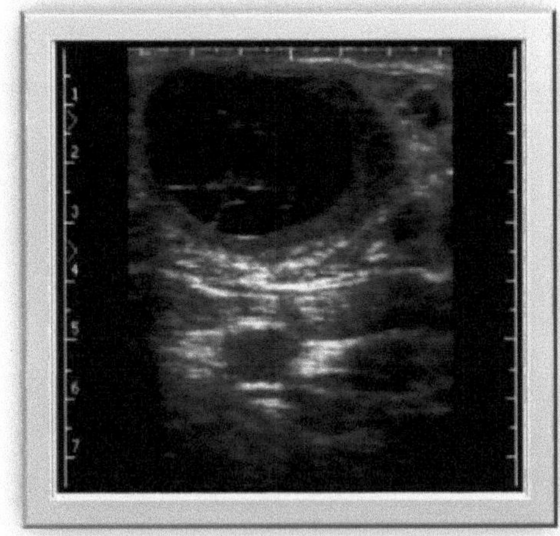

Figure 32. Luteal cyst - Ultrasound image. Anechoic cavity > 25 mm - Wall > 3 mm

Fibrinous trabeculae Photo: Reproduction Unit, ENVT. Linear endorectal probe TRINGA® Linear -ESAOTE ultrasound scanner [Dornier P and Droui X (2013)]

1.4.1.3.2 Yellow body

In bovine gynaecology, the presence of the corpus luteum is systematically sought. It is used to determine whether the female has cycled and to assess the development of the corpus luteum in order to rationalise the use of PGF2α. When diagnosing gestation, it is used to guide the search for the conceptus in the horn ipsilateral to the corpus luteum. The mature corpus luteum, spherical or "champagne cork" in shape, is hypoechoic compared with the ovarian parenchyma due to non-specular reflections (ultrasound image 7). It appears as a homogeneous, well-defined grey structure, and may have a more echogenic line in the centre corresponding to denser fibrous tissue. The diameter of the mature corpus luteum is greater than 2 cm. Around 40% of mature corpora lutea have a central cavity less than 2 cm in diameter containing anechoic fluid. These cavitated corpora lutea are considered to be normal luteal structures. (See Figures 35, 36, 37 and 38).

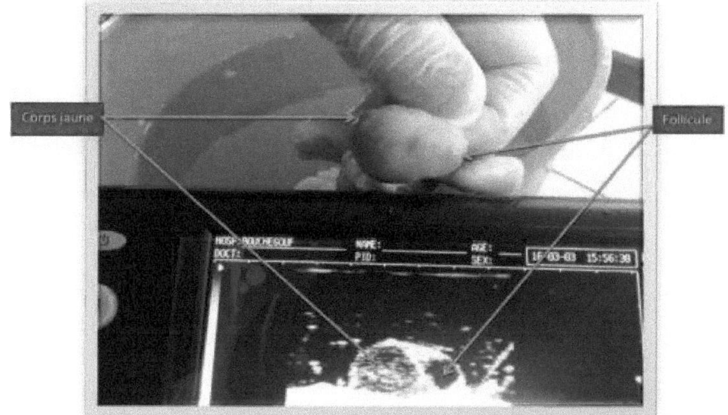

Figure 33. Ultrasound image of ovary showing corpus luteum and follicle (Original photo 2016)

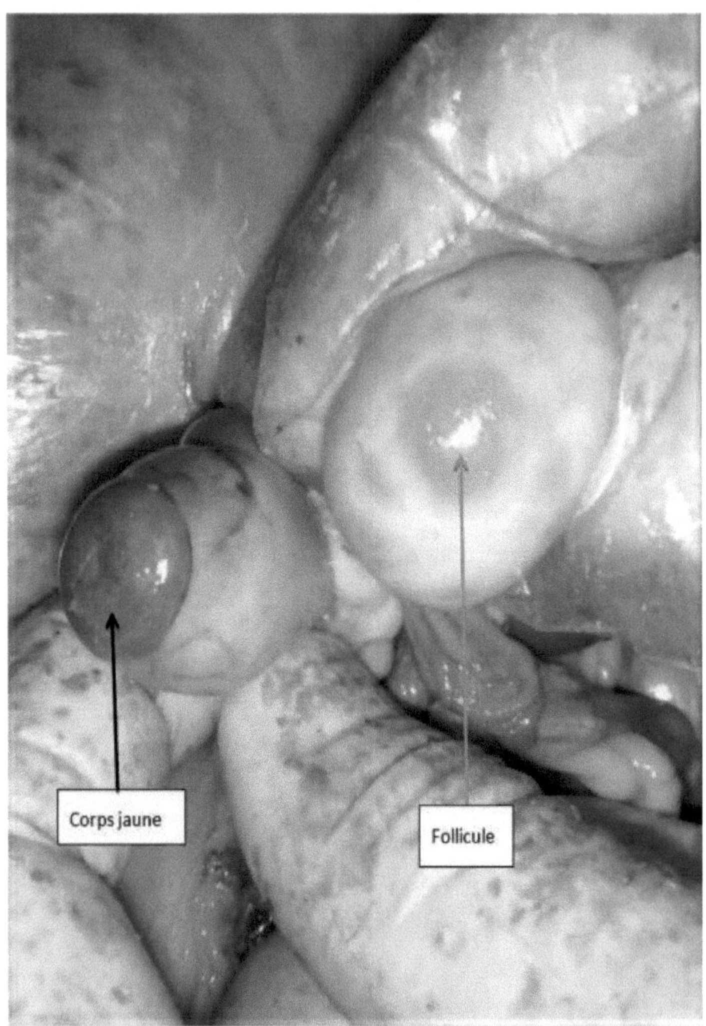

Figure 34. Corpus luteum and follicle. (Original photo 2016)

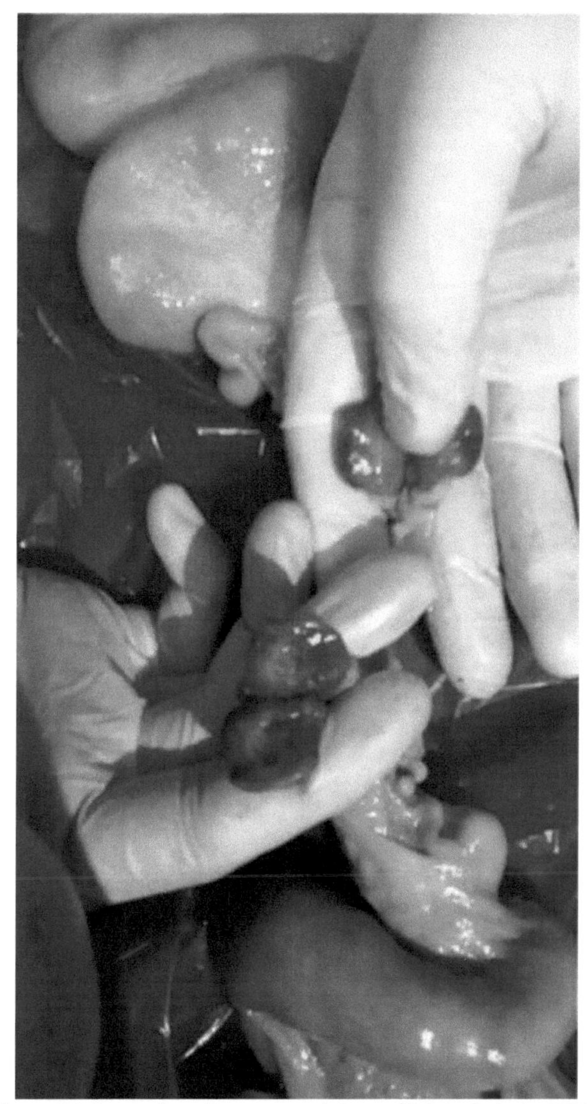

Figure 35. Severed cavitary corpus luteum (Original photo 2016)

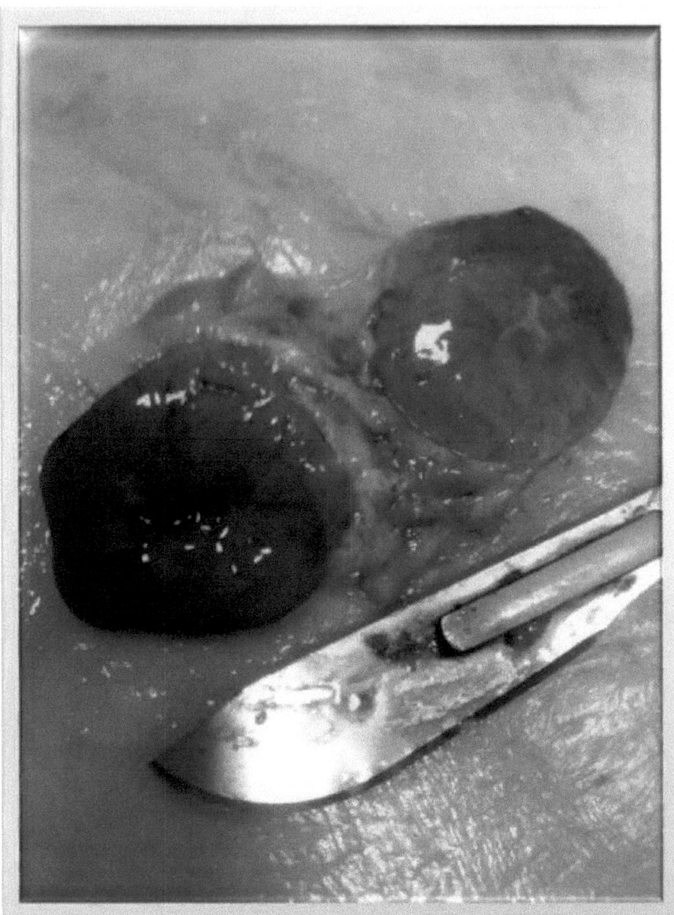

Figure 36. Yellow body (Original photo 2016)

1.4.1.3.3 The uterus

The body of the bovine uterus is short (3 cm long) and is extended by two long horns (30 to 40 cm) connected at their bifurcation by two intercornuate ligaments. The diameter of the horns at the base varies from 2 to 4 cm and gradually decreases to 5-6 mm at the utero-tubal junction. The way they are curved can be compared to the shape of a racing bike handlebar. The walls of the uterus are made up of a mucous layer rich in glands (endometrium), a powerful muscular layer (myometrium) and a serosa. A linear probe applied dorsally to the uterus provides a longitudinal section of the organ, with its great curvature forming a convex curve. In most cases, it is difficult to see the entire curvature of a uterine horn in a single cutting plane, but the horn is cut in several places. The section of the uterine wall appears in grey tones and with a variable granular structure. On a transverse or longitudinal section, a hyperechoic zone appears at the periphery of the uterine horn, corresponding to the myometrium, while a weakly echogenic zone is observed close to the lumen, corresponding to the endometrium (See Figure 39).

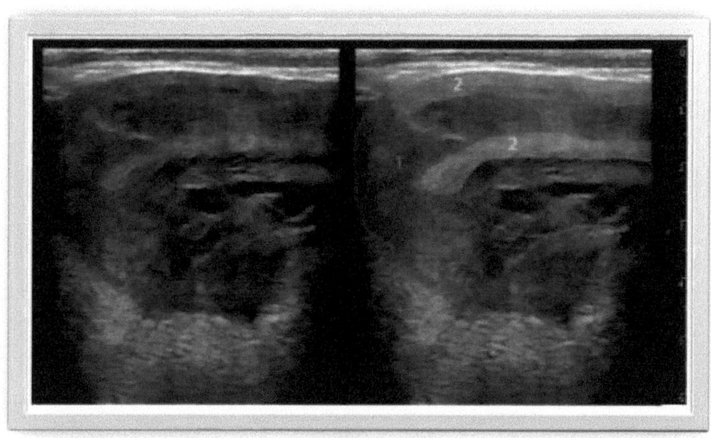

Figure 37. Longitudinal section of a uterine horn in the peri-oestrous period
1: Uterine horn in longitudinal section - 2: Hyperechoic areas (myometrium) - 3: Broad ligament (Scale: one scale corresponds to 0.5 cm) (Taveau and Julia 2013).

1.4.2 Ultrasound examination of the pregnant genital tract

There are various techniques for diagnosing pregnancy, such as transrectal palpation, tests for pregnancy indicators (progesterone, zygotin, PAG (Pregnancy Associated Proteins) or oestrogen) and ultrasound, which can also offer a number of advantages, especially in the absence of other diagnostic methods:

- Mobile, ready to use at any time and easy to handle
- early diagnosis: diagnosis can be made as early as 25-30 days gestation
- Reliability: ultrasound diagnosis of pregnancy has a sensitivity of 97.7% and a specificity of 87.7% between 26 and 33 days' gestation. Sensitivity can be as high as 100% from day 29 ^{e}.
- safety: early pregnancy diagnosis by ultrasound does not increase the embryonic mortality rate.
- speed: the diagnosis is made directly on the farm, at the animal's bedside. However, the purchase of an ultrasound scanner is still a major investment, and its use requires a certain amount of training to improve the reliability of diagnoses.

1.4.2.1 Reminder of the stages of embryonic development

In the cow, the embryo at the morula stage arrives in the uterine cavity 4 days after fertilisation and measures one tenth of a millimetre (see Figure 40). At 9^{e} days, it loses its spheroid shape and reaches a diameter of 0.2 mm, growing in length: the diameter of the embryonic vesicle remains constant, at 2 mm on average, between 12^{e} and 20^{e} days. The filamentous blastocyst completely invades the horn ipsilateral to the corpus luteum on day 17^{e} and the contralateral horn between day 20^{e} and day 32^{e} of gestation; this phase corresponds to elongation. Implantation of the conceptus begins on day 19^{e} of gestation (see Figure 41). The term embryo is used in the first 42 days of gestation, and foetus beyond this date (See Figures N° 42 and 43). Diagnosis of gestation can be made from 25^{e} days after insemination. Before this, the embryonic vesicle does not exceed a few millimetres, so it is very difficult to observe by ultrasound.

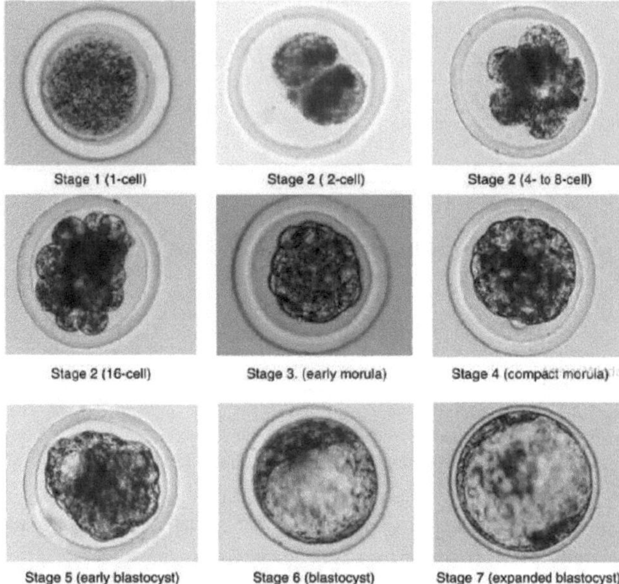

Figure 40: Early days of bovine embryo development

(Photos Brad Lindsey by Marianna. Source: https://veteriankey.com 2017)

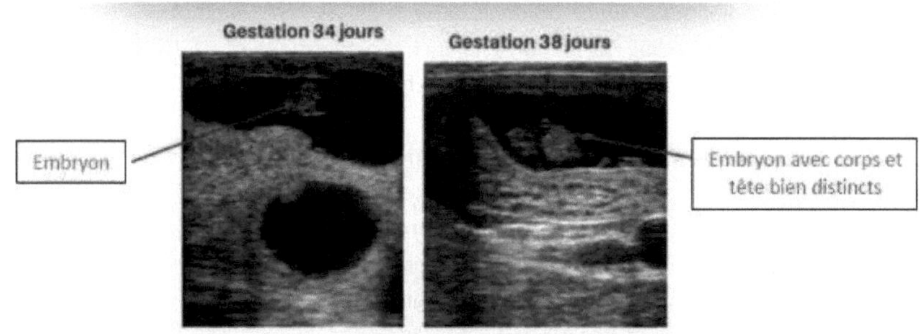

Figure 38. Embryos aged 34 and 38 days

(Photo Thierry Vernoux 2021. Source: https://www.web-agri.fr)

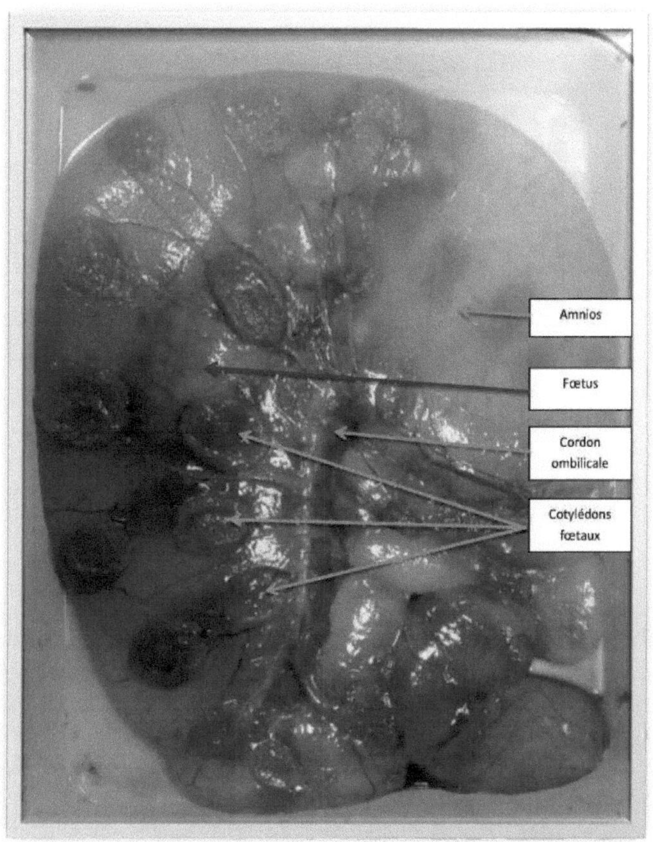

Figure 39. Cattle placenta (Original photos 2016)

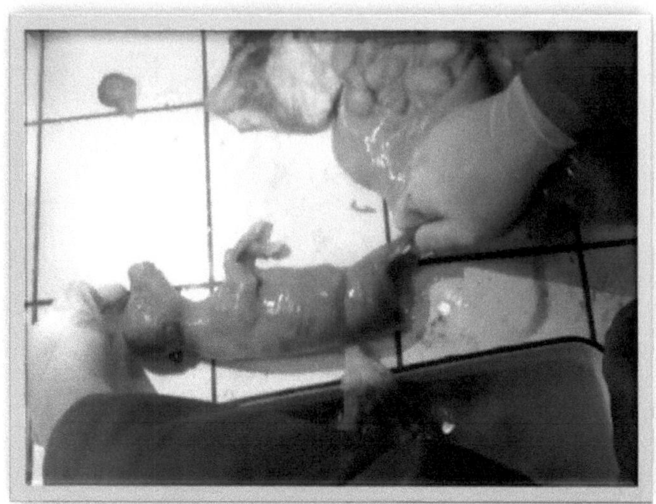

Figure 40. 05-month-old bovine foetus (Original photos 2016)

1.4.3 Diagnosis of early gestation

Diagnosing early gestation is a more or less straightforward examination, depending on the age of the animal, the position of the genital tract, the breed and the veterinarian's experience. It is most accurate when the conceptus is visualised. By day 25^{e} , the embryonic vesicle is 10 mm in diameter and the 8-9 mm long embryo is pressed against the uterine wall. Ultrasound can then show the presence of fluid in the uterine horns, as well as the vesicle often present in the free part of the horns 2.

Between day 25^{e} and day 30^{e} , the embryo can be seen as a clear spot in a fluid sac, often pressed against the uterine wall. It is sometimes hidden by a uterine fold and is therefore difficult to visualise. (See Figure 44).

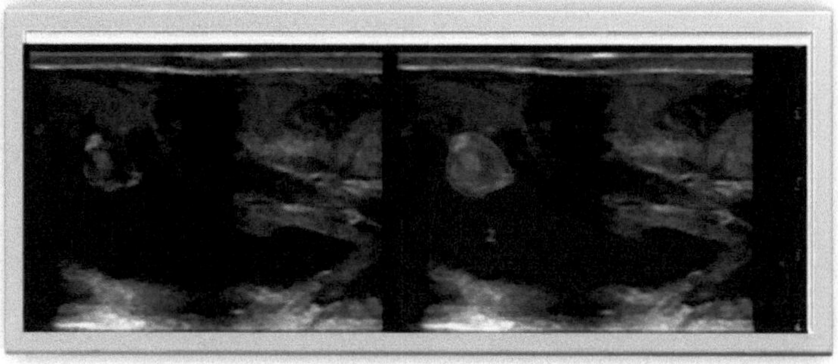

Figure 41. Ultrasound image 29-day gestation

1 1: embryo - 2: uterine lumen containing conceptus fluid

(Scale: one scale corresponds to 0.5 cm) (Taveau and Julia 2013).

After 30 days of gestation, the diameter of the allantoic vesicle increases rapidly (the vesicle subsequently fuses with the chorion to form the allantochorion). It contains the amnion, the innermost foetal membrane delimiting the amniotic cavity in which the embryo bathes. At the same time, the embryo grows by around 1 mm per day between days 25^{e} and 50^{e} of gestation. From day 30e , it is possible to visualise the amniotic membrane in the form of a fine echogenic line, then at day 40e it is possible to identify the attachment of the umbilical cord and the various organs, this end of organogenesis marks the transition to the foetal stage.

From 45-50ème days, the first ossification centres can be seen on the foetus in the ribs, vertebrae, pelvis, skull, etc. The placentomes, a placental unit consisting of the foetal cotyledon (chorionic valve) and the maternal wattle, are visible close to the embryo from day 35e (see Figure 21). To ensure the viability of the conceptus, the beating of the embryonic heart is observed from day 25^{e} of gestation. From day 45^{e} onwards, it is also important to pay attention to foetal movements, the appearance of the foetal fluid, which must be homogeneous, anechogenic and in sufficient quantity, and the development and integrity of the foetus (see Figure 45).

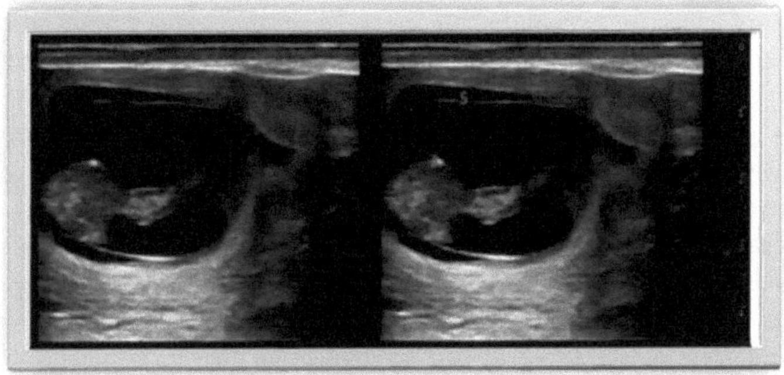

Figure 42. Fetus at 50 days gestation - transverse section

2 2: body; 3: limb outlines; 4: umbilical cord; 5: amnion (Scale: one graduation corresponds to 0.5 cm) (Taveau and Julia 2013).

In practice, ultrasound examination allows early diagnosis of pregnancy from 28^{e}

- 30^{e} day post insemination. This examination is based on 3 main criteria:
- the presence of liquid in the horns (in the form of anechoic areas)
- identification of the embryo measuring just a few millimetres
- examining its viability by visualising its heartbeat.

The diagnosis of late gestation is made after 100 days' gestation. At this stage, transrectal ultrasound is of limited use, as the foetus and changes to the uterus can be detected by transrectal palpation. From the 4th to 5th month of gestation, the fetus's considerable weight drags it downwards and it becomes difficult to explore it using transrectal ultrasound. Abdominal ultrasound from the right flank can then be considered, but is of limited use in practice (Figure 46).

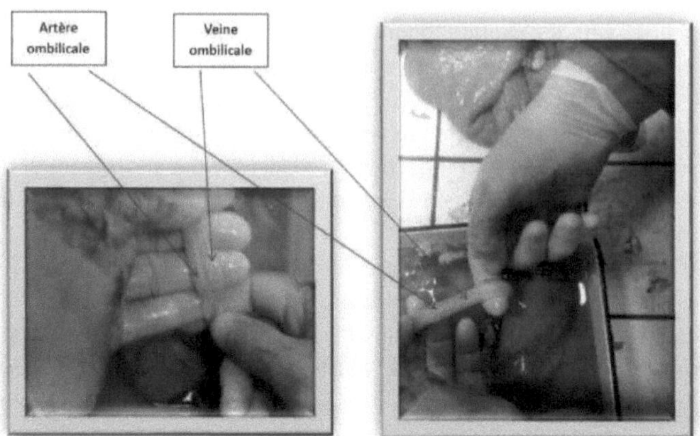

Figure 43. Umbilical cord (bovine foetus over 100 days old) (Original photo 2016)

1.4.4 Diagnosis of non-pregnancy

The diagnosis of non-pregnancy usually requires a longer examination. To establish this diagnosis, it is important to look for the presence or absence of corpus luteum on the ovaries (to be differentiated from cyclical corpus luteum and persistent corpus luteum). The absence of a corpus luteum supports the diagnosis of non-pregnancy. If there is no corpus luteum, the entire uterus should be examined in detail, and the horn ipsilateral to the corpus luteum should be checked for the absence of fluid.

1.4.5 Diagnosis of foetal sex

This diagnosis is primarily of economic interest, as it can be used, for example, to increase the value of the sale of pregnant cows carrying a female foetus, to adapt the decisions to be taken in the event of dystocic parturition, or to plan the management of herd renewal. Sex diagnosis in bovine gynaecology was first established in 1986 by identifying the external genitalia (scrotum, penis, teats) between days 70^{e} and 120^{e} of gestation. Although reliable, this technique is rarely used nowadays, in favour of early sexing, which aims to locate the genital tubercle between 55 and 65 days gestation. This method, described for the first time in 1989 by Curran et al. Initially located halfway between the tail and the umbilical cord (up to the 50-day stage), the genital tubercle migrates towards the umbilical cord in males and becomes the penis, while in females it migrates towards the tail, evolving into the clitoris. This migration is considered complete at 55 days gestation.

In both sexes, the genital tubercle is a bilobed hyperechoic structure. The main risks of error when diagnosing sex are due to confusion of the tubercle with neighbouring structures (the tail when identifying a female foetus, the umbilical cord for a male foetus), as well as confusion between the body of the penis and the median raphe of the female, or misorientation of the foetus which can lead to confusion between sections of the limbs and the genital tubercle.

In order to make this diagnosis, it is important to make the appropriate cross-sections according to the foetal structures identified (head, limbs, umbilical cord, etc.). Sex diagnosis is carried out using transverse sections or a horizontal section, in order to clearly visualise the structures of interest. Sagittal sections are not suitable for sex diagnosis. In practice, this examination requires considerable experience, as intermediate sections are often obtained due to the mobility of the foetus.

In practice, after orienting the foetus on transverse sections, the genital tubercle is sought between the umbilical cord and the tail. In the case of a female diagnosis, it is important to check that there is no genital tubercle behind the cord, in addition to identifying the genital tubercle in a posterior position, under the tail. Horizontal sections allow all the structures of interest (limb sections, umbilical cord, tail section and genital bud) to be visualised on the same image, taken on the ventral edge of the abdomen (Figure No. 47).

After 70 days, the genital tubercle is covered by the labia minora or prepuce, so it loses its echogenicity and bilobed appearance and becomes less visible on ultrasound. At the same time, the external genitalia (scrotum, udders) become visible and will serve as a basis for diagnosing the sex of the foetus. In females, the teats are visible from 70 days, appearing as four hyperechoic points, arranged in a diamond shape between the hindquarters.

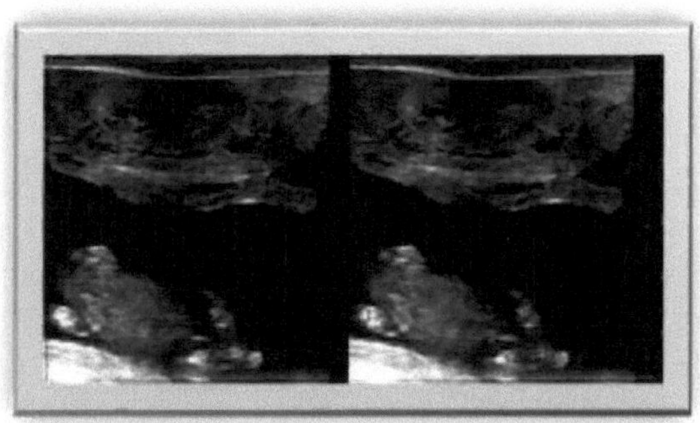

Figure 44. Female foetus at 58 days gestation - horizontal section

1: limbs; 2: tail; 3: median raphe; 4: genital tubercle. (Scale: one scale corresponds to 0.5 cm) (Taveau and Julia 2013)

In the male, the scrotum, a two-lobed mass in the middle of the pelvic region, and the penis, a bulge behind the umbilical cord, can be seen (see Figure 48). The more advanced the stage of gestation, the more difficult it will be to diagnose the sex of the foetus, due to its large size and the difficulty of locating the topography on the ultrasound screen. In addition, the fetus is less and less accessible due to its location in the abdominal cavity. It is therefore recommended that late sex diagnosis be carried out between 80 and 100 days gestation.

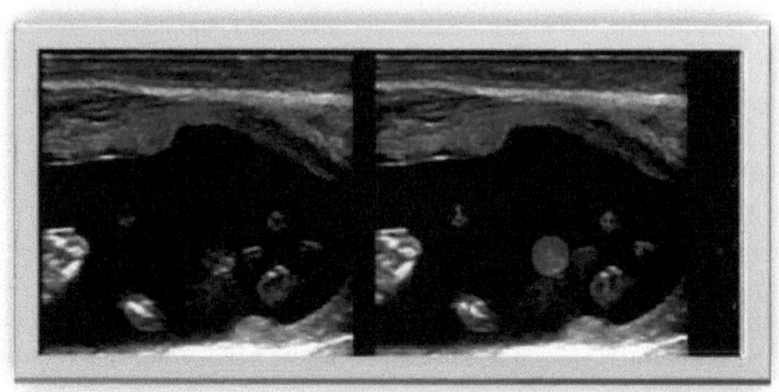

Figure 45. Male foetus at 58 days gestation - horizontal section

1: limbs; 2: tail; 3: median raphe; 4: genital tubercle. (Scale: one scale corresponds to 0.5 cm) (Taveau and Julia 2013)

1.4.6 Diagnosis of twin boys

Twin gestation is taking on an interesting role in bovine reproduction for technical purposes in the monitoring of cattle breeding and above all to take all precautions due to the possibility of complications arising during parturition. In fact, studies show that twin gestation increases the mortality rate of calves compared to those born from a single gestation. In practice, this diagnosis requires observation of both embryos on the same section to avoid any misinterpretation, which makes it difficult to carry out. For this reason, it is imperative to examine both ovaries first, looking for the presence of more than one corpus luteum, before carefully examining both horns. The most favourable period for detecting twins is between 30 and 100 days gestation, with an optimum between 40 and 75 days (see Figure 49).

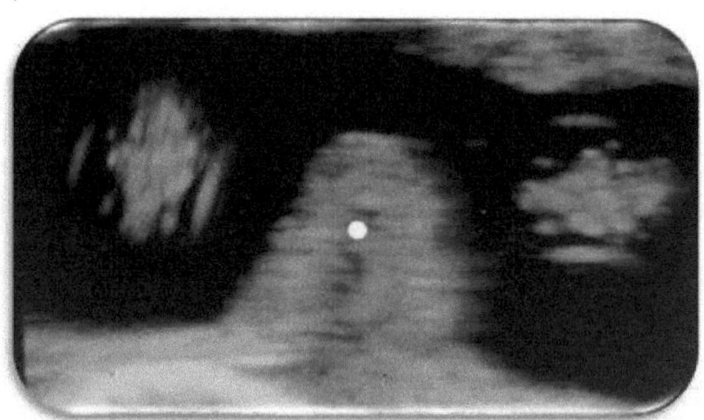

Figure 46. Twin gestation

(Photos Beausoleil Lauson. Source: https://www.laterre.ca 2021)

1.4.7 Diagnosis of gestational pathologies

1.4.7.1 Uterine pathologies

1.4.7.1.1 Endometritis or metritis

Endometritis or metritis is inflammation of the uterus, generally of infectious origin. There are several types, and metritis occurs after parturition during the first 21 days. It is characterised by general symptoms (anorexia, hyperthermia) and local symptoms (purulent vaginal discharge). Endometritis is characterised by abnormal genital discharge, ranging from cloudy mucus to pus, and by the absence of general symptoms. Pyometra is the accumulation of pus in the uterine cavity, associated with a persistent corpus luteum and closure of the uterine cervix (not to be confused with gestation on rectal palpation). It is easy to detect on ultrasound examination. The ultrasound image is characterised by the presence of heterogeneous uterine contents with a flaky appearance. Clumps of suspended pus can be mobilised by suctioning the uterus. In this case, a corpus luteum may also be present (see Figure 50). Subclinical endometritis is often encountered and is accompanied by the presence of an inflammatory state of the endometrium and characterised by the absence of abnormal genital secretions observed on vaginoscopic examination. It is characterised by a minimal amount of exudate in the uterine cavity and the presence of neutrophils in the uterine lumen, and is therefore not clinically detectable without further examination (cytology). This makes it virtually impossible to diagnose by ultrasound. On the other hand, ultrasound can in some cases detect certain endometritis by showing uterine fluids with echogenic particles in suspension. The ease of diagnosis depends on the quantity of fluid present and therefore the degree of endometritis. For example, an anechogenic zone can be seen in the cranial part of the uterus, with the uterus sloping downwards and most often presenting a star shape (see Figure 51). However, ultrasound diagnosis leads to an overestimate of cows with endometritis, as there are several situations other than endometritis associated with the presence of fluid in the uterus, for which cytological examination is recommended.

Ultrasound examination should therefore be used to make a differential diagnosis with oestrus, early gestation or embryonic death. Ultrasound only supports the history and other examinations (transrectal palpation, vaginal examination of uterine secretions or bacteriology).

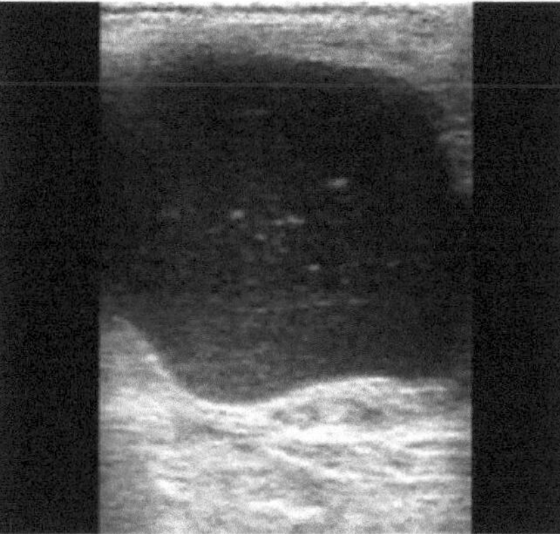

Figure 50. ultrasound image of a pyometra (heterogeneous uterine content)
(Photo Hanzen FMV Liège)

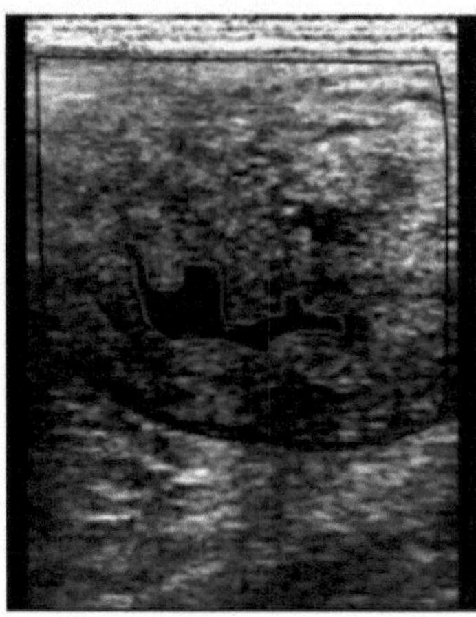

Figure 47. Ultrasound image of chronic endometritis (the blue line identifies the outline of the uterine wall and the red line the outline of the uterine cavity in a star shape).
(Photo Hanzen FMV Liège)

1.4.7.1.2 Hydrosalpinx

Hydrosalpinx, as its name suggests, corresponds to a collection of serous fluid (hydric) accumulating in the uterine tube, also known as the oviduct or salpinx, which is a flexible cord, 10 to 15 cm long and with a sinuous course (See Figures N° 52). Its presence is always abnormal; the hydrosalpinx appears on ultrasound as anechoic circular images, often circumscribed close to the ovary (See Figures N° 53). These are known as "balloon-like" images. It is important to differentiate this from early gestation, taking into account topographical landmarks.

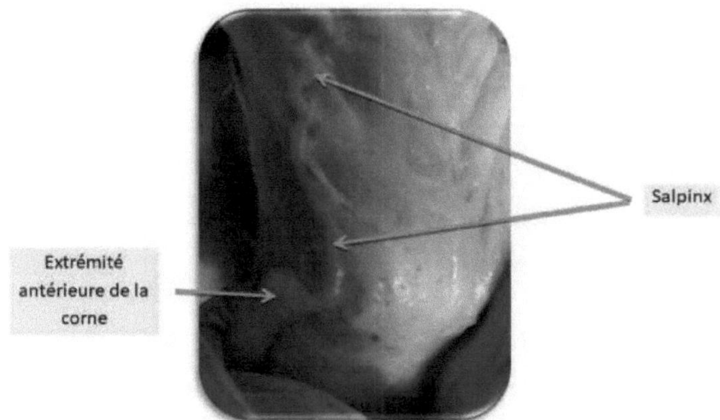

Figure 52. Uterine tube (Oviduct or Salpinx) (Original photo 2018)

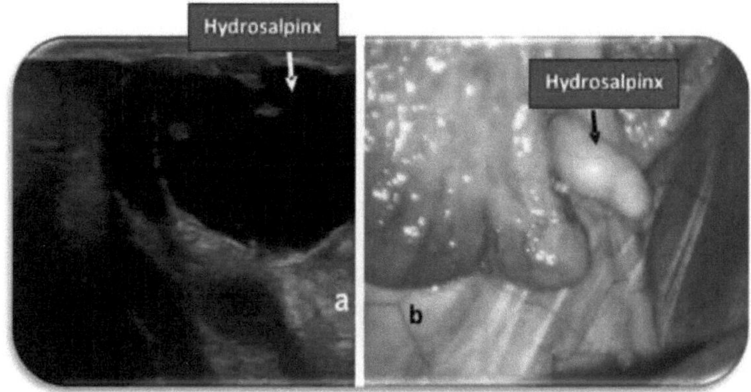

Figure 53. Hydrosalpinx (arrow). (a) Ultrasound image (b) Laparoscopic image

(Photo Khursheed and Madhumeet 2018)

1.4.7.1.3 Ovarian tumours

Granulosa tumours are the most common ovarian tumours. However, they are rare in cows, with an incidence of less than 0.5%. They can lead to changes in behaviour (an oestrus or nymphomania) and should be suspected when the ovary is larger than 10 cm.

Their structure and size vary greatly from case to case. On ultrasound, the echogenicity is generally heterogeneous, with multiple anechogenic cavities corresponding to follicles or blood vessels.

1.4.7.1.4 Embryonic and foetal mortality

Embryonic mortality means the interruption of gestation during the stage of embryonic life from fertilisation to 42^{e} days, which corresponds to the end of organogenesis. Beyond 42 days, we speak of foetal mortality. Embryonic mortality, which is more difficult to detect, can be divided into two periods:

- Early embryonic death which takes place before maternal recognition of gestation and which occurs before the embryonic signal (trophoblast) is emitted, the 15^{e} - 17^{e} days of gestation, i.e. generally before the completion of a cycle or in other words in this case the return to heat is not delayed in relation to the length of the cycle.
- Late embryonic mortality which occurs after maternal recognition (16 days) and on day 42^{e} of gestation, and which is associated with a delayed return to heat, beyond 25 days.

Most embryonic deaths occur before 25^{e} days gestation, although the period between 25^{e} and 42^{e} days gestation is critical, as it corresponds to implantation.

The diagnosis of embryonic and foetal mortality on ultrasound is established during sequential examinations by the demonstration of an embryo at one moment and the absence of an embryo or foetus a little later (or a return to heat) (See Figure N° 54). In real time, the diagnosis of this pathology of gestation is based on several criteria such as the size of the foetus being reduced in relation to the stage of gestation, the structures observed are difficult to interpret and the finding of numerous echogenic debris in the amniotic or allantoic fluid is the rule. It is therefore important and advisable to look for signs of vitality in the embryo or foetus (heartbeat, movements, etc.). If in doubt, it is best to repeat the ultrasound examination.

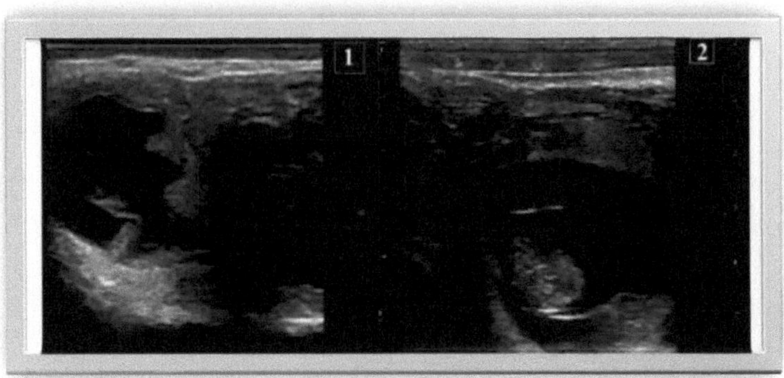

Figure 54. Comparison of two pregnancies at 42 days

1: embryonic mortality; 2: physiological gestation

The amnion and the foetus in cross-section are clearly visible in image 2, whereas the structures of the conceptus are more blurred on image 1. (Scale: one scale corresponds to 1 cm on the left image, and 0.5 cm on the right image).

(Taveau and Julia 2013)

1.4.7.1.5 Foetal mummification or maceration

Mummification is in fact an aseptic transformation of the foetus, characterised by the resorption of the allantoic and amniotic fluids, the placenta detaches and attaches itself to the foetus. The muscles retract, the skin autolyses and the foetus is transformed into a brownish, slimy mass which may undergo calcareous infiltration, justifying the name *lithopedion* sometimes given to the mummified foetus (see Figure 55).

Unlike mummification, maceration is caused by bacterial digestion of the foetus, characterised by slow impregnation of its tissues by body fluids, leading to their softening and dissolution. The bones separate and end up bathed in a yellowish liquid mass with no stench. These liquids can sometimes reabsorb and some settle in the uterine wall.

The diagnosis of foetal mummification is established when the ultrasound images show a mass of hyperechoic intrauterine tissue without fluid, a cluster of hyperechoic bone with shadow cones, sometimes associated with a thickened uterine wall.

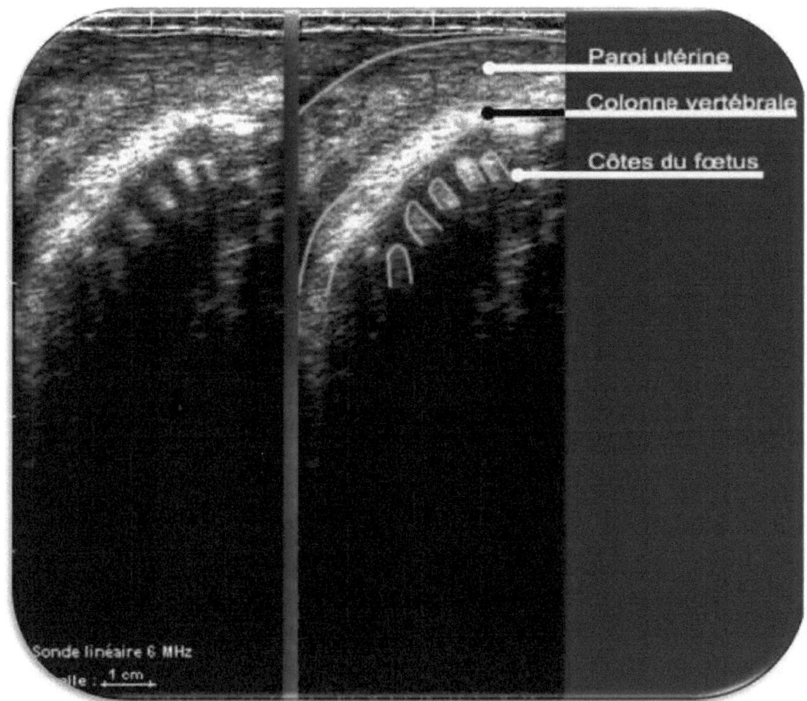

Figure 55. Mummified foetus
(Photo Calais and Dreno 2004)

Conclusion

The management of reproduction and breeding in the bovine species, and more specifically in breeding and milk production farms, is a very important and onerous veterinary task, since it requires clinicians to acquire a solid training in the speciality, enabling them to choose the best treatment for each clinical case presented, following the establishment of a good diagnosis based on a better aetiological knowledge during the performance of a clinical examination of the cow's genital tract that is well adapted and well managed. This book has been written with this in mind, and I hope that it will help and contribute to the reinforcement of skills in the field of reproductive pathology and thus to the development of the veterinarian's performance.

BIBLIOGRAPHICAL REFERENCES

[01]. **ACHEMAOUI A.a, BENDAHMANE M.b**, (2015). Analysis of reproduction parameters in a private dairy cattle farm in the wilaya of Sidi Bel Abbés. Revue " Nature & Technologie ". B- Sciences Agronomiques et Biologiques, n° 14/ Janvier 2016, Pages 20 à 22.

[02]. **ADAMS G, BOLLWEIN H, BUCZINSKI S, CARRIERE PD, CHASTANT-MAILLARD S, COLLOTON J, CRUVINEL HMR, CURRAN S, DESCÔTEAUX L, DUROCHER J,GAYRARD V, GNEMMI G, GONZALES-BULMES A, LEFEBVRE R, MARTIN GB, MATSUI M, MIYAMOTO A, PARRAGUEZ H, PICARD-HAGEN N, RAGGI LA, RATTO M, SALE S, SALES ZLATAR F, STROUD B, VINOLES-GIL C** (2009). Guide pratique d'échographie pour la reproduction des ruminants. Paris: Med'com. 239 p. ISBN 978-2-35403-028-5.

[03]. **ALVES DE OLIVIERA L, AUBRY P, BADINAND F, BAREILLE N, BERTHELOT X, BOUCHARDE, BOUSQUET D, BRODEUR M, BUCZINSKI S, CARRIERE PD, CHANVAILLON A, CHASTANTS, COLLOTON J, DESCÔTEAUX L, DISENHAUS C, DORE M, DUBUC C, ENJALBERT F, GAYRARD V, HANZEN C, HARVEY D, LEFEBVRE R, NOUVEL X, OPSONER G, PICARDHAGEN N, ROY JP, SEEGERS H, STOCK A, TAINTURIER D, VAILLANCOURT D** (2012). VADE-MECUM of reproductive management of dairy cattle in the bovine species. *Annales de Médecine Vétérinaire*, 151, 247-256. Paris: Med'com. 240 p. ISBN : 978-2-35-403-093-3.

[04]. **BARR F, GASCHEN L** (2011). *BSAVA manual of canine and feline ultrasonography*. England: BSAVA. 222 p. ISBN 978-1-905319-30-5.

[05]. **BOUAZIZ O.** Pathology of the uterus (2012). El-khroub Institute of Veterinary Sciences, Constantine.

[06]. **BUDRAS KD, HABEL RE, WÜNSCHE A, BUDA S, JAHRMÄRKER G, RICHTER R, STARKE D** (2003). *Bovine Anatomy: An illustrated text*. First edition. Hannover, Germany: Schlütersche. 138 p. ISBN 3-89993-000-2.

[07]. **CALAIS E.I.M, DRENO C.M** (2004). L'ECHOGRAPHIE EN GYNECOLOGIE BOVINE, OVINE ET CAPRINE : REALISATION D'UN CD-ROM DIDACTIQUE. Doctoral thesis in veterinary medicine, Faculté de Médecine de Créteil.

[08]. **DEGUILLAUME L** (2010). Post-partum genital inflammation in cows. University thesis, AgroparisTech, 206 p.

[09]. **DEGUILLAUME L, CHASTANT-MAILLARD S** (2009). How to diagnose endometritis in cows. Bulletin des GTV, 49, 101-105.

[10]. **DORNIER P, DROUI X** (2013). Follicular cysts in dairy cows: ultrasound evaluation of the efficacy of progestin treatment and relationship with genital inflammation. Thesis to obtain the grade of veterinary doctor (Toulouse National Veterinary School).

[11]. **EDMONDSON AJ, FISSORE RA, PASHEN RL, BONDURNT RH** (1986). The use of ultrasonography for the study of the bovine reproductive tract I. Normal and pathological ovarian structures. Animal Reproduction Science, 12, 157-165.

[12]. **FIENI F, TAINTURUER D, BRUYAS JF, BATTUT I** (1998). Echotomographic examination of the ovaries in cows. Journées nationales des GTV, Tours 27, 28 et 29 mai 1998, 411415.

[13]. **FISSORE RA, EDMONSON AJ, PASHEN RL, BONDURANT RH** (1986). The use of ultrasonography for the study of the bovine reproductive tract II. Non-pregnant, pregnant and pathological conditions of the uterus. Animal Reproduction Science, 12, 167-177.

[14]. **HAGEN et al.** Reproductive Pathology 2016. 109, 35-44.

[15]. **HANZEN C.** (2014). Obstetrics : The pharmacological control of parturition in ruminants (Université de Liège, VETE0443-1 Thériogénologie des animaux de production).

[16]. **HANZEN C.** (2014). Obstetrics : Obstetrical complications in ruminants (Université de Liège, VETE0443-1 Thériogénologie des animaux de production).

[17]. **HANZEN C.** (2014). Obstetrics : Dystocies in ruminants (Université de Liège, VETE0443-1 Thériogénologie des animaux de production)

[18]. **HANZEN C.** (2014). Obstetrics : Obstetrical interventions in ruminants (Université de Liège, VETE0443-1 Thériogénologie des animaux de production).
[19]. **HANZEN C.** (2014). Pathologie : La maîtrise des cycles chez les petits ruminants (Université de Liège, VETE0443-1 Thériogénologie des animaux de production).
[20]. **HANZEN C.** (2014). Pathologies: An epidemiological approach to bovine reproduction. Reproduction management (University of Liège, VETE0492 Herd medicine).
[21]. **HANZEN C.** (2014). Pathologies: Pubertal and postpartum anestrus in the bovine species (Université de Liège, VETE0443-1 Thériogénologie des animaux de production).
[22]. **HANZEN C.** (2014). Pathologies: Uterine involution and delayed uterine involution in cows (Université de Liège, VETE0443-1 Thériogénologie des animaux de production).
[23]. **HANZEN C.** (2014). Pathologies: Placental retention in cows (Université de Liège, VETE0443-1 Thériogénologie des animaux de production).
[24]. **HANZEN C.** (2014). Pathologies: Infertility and infertility factors in bovine reproduction (Université de Liège, VETE0443-1 Thériogénologie des animaux de production).
[25]. **HANZEN C.** (2014). Pathologies: Uterine infections in cows (Université de Liège, VETE0443-1 Thériogénologie des animaux de production).
[26]. **HANZEN C.** (2014). Pathologies: Ovarian cysts in cows (Université de Liège, VETE0443-1 Thériogénologie des animaux de production).
[27]. **HANZEN C.** (2014). Pathologies: Pathologies of the female genital tract of ruminants (Université de Liège, VETE0443-1 Thériogénologie des animaux de production).
[28]. **HANZEN C.** (2014). Semiology: applications of ultrasound to ruminant reproduction (VETE0443-1 Theriogenology of production animals).
[29]. **HANZEN C.** (2014). Semiology : The detection of estrus in ruminants (Université de Liège, VETE0448-1 Sémiologie des animaux de production).
[30]. **HANZEN C.** (2014). Semiology : The propaedeutics of the female genital tract of ruminants (Université de Liège, VETE0448-1 Sémiologie des animaux de production).
[31]. **HANZEN C.** (2014). Sémiologie : Le constat de gestation chez les ruminants (Université de Liège, VETE0448-1 Sémiologie des animaux de production).
[32]. **HANZEN C.** (2014). Obstetrical semiology : The obstetrical propaedeutic of ruminants (Université de Liège, VETE0448-1 Sémiologie des animaux de production).
[33]. **HANZEN C,** BASCON F, THERON L, LOPEZ-GATIUS F (2007). Ovarian cysts
[34]. **https://www.**laterre.ca/chroniques/page-conseils/gestation-de-jumeaux-en production-dairy-2nd-part/ (2020).
[35]. **https://www.**web-agri.fr/reproduction/article/181480/echographier-ses-vaches-allaitantes-soi-meme (2021). Ultrasound by the farmer: Identifying pregnant cows to manage suckler culls.
[36]. **JAUDON JP, PERROT C, VIAUD F, CADORE J** (1991). Physical, technological and semiological bases of medical ultrasonography. *Point Vétérinaire*, 23 (135), 11-18.
[37]. **KÄHN W** (1994). Atlas de diagnostics échographiques. Paris: Maloine. 255 p. ISBN: 2 224-02282-4.
[38]. **KAMIMURA S, OHGI T, TAKAHASHI M, TSUKAMOTO T** (1993). Postpartum resumption of ovarian activity and uterine involution monitored by ultrasonography in Holstein cows. The Journal of Veterinary Medicine Science, 55, 643-647.
[39]. **KHURSHEED AS, MADHUMEET S, (2018).** Ultrasonography and laparoscopy as a diagnostic tool for evaluation of genitalia in cows. The Indian journal of animal sciences. DOI: 10.56093/ijans.v88i11.85030.
[40]. **LEBASTARD D.** (1997) Echography in bovine gynaecology: possible uses in rural practice. Le Point Vétérinaire, 28, (181), 1089-1096.
[41]. **Marianna M. Jahnke, James K. West and Curtis R. Youngs** (2017). Evaluation of In

Vivo- Derived Bovine Embryos. https://veteriankey.com/evaluation-of-in-vivo-derived-bovine-embryos/.
[42]. **MARTINAT-BOTTE F, RENAUD G, MADEC F, COSTIOU P, TERQUI M** (1998). The principle of ultrasound. In Echographie et reproduction chez la truie : bases et applications pratiques. Paris : INRA, p. 10-15.
[43]. **MULLER E, WITTKOWSKI G** (1986). Visualization of male and female characteristics of bovine fetuses by real-time ultrasonic. Theriogenology, 25, (4), 571-574.
[44]. **PAUZAC F.** (1875). La dystocie chez la vache, thesis for the diploma of veterinary surgeon. (École Nationale Vétérinaire de Toulouse). reproduction in cattle. *Revue de Médecine Vétérinaire*, 167, (1), 21-31.
[45]. **SINGH J, PIERSON RA, ADAMS GP** (1997). Ultrasound image attributes of the bovine corpus luteum: structural and functional correlates. Journal of Reproduction and Fertility, 109, 35-44.
[46]. **STEENHOLDT CW** (1997). Chapter 48 - Infertility Due to Non-inflammatory Abnormalities of the Tubular Reproductive Tract. Pages 294 - 303. In: Current therapy in large animal theriogenology. First edition. Philadelphia: W.B. Saunders Company. P.1033-1061.
[47]. **TAVEAU J, JULIA J** (2013). Physiology and pathology of cow reproduction: Development of online teaching resources based on ultrasound images of the reproductive system. THESIS FOR THE DIPLOMA OF VETERINARY PHYSICIAN (Université Paul Sabatier de Toulouse).

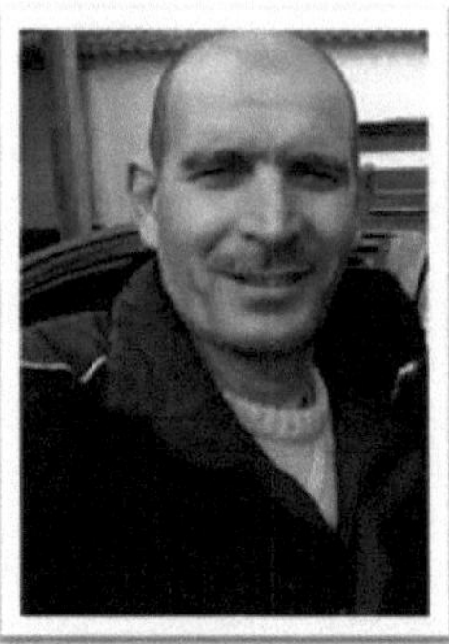

Born on 25.03.1966 in Khenchela (Algeria), Dr Zeroual Fayçal studied veterinary science at the University of Constantine, where he obtained his Doctorate in Veterinary Medicine in June 1992.

He practised as a veterinary surgeon for twenty years (1992-2013), during which time he acquired and perfected his knowledge and skills in the field, particularly in the monitoring of ruminant breeding and reproduction. He is regarded as a pioneer in the field of improving cattle breeds through artificial insemination programmes.

In addition to his veterinary career, the author has also been involved in teaching veterinary science at university since 1993. After working for many years as an associate lecturer at UCBET (formerly the Institut Agro-Vétérinaire de l'Université d'Annaba), he returned to the university in 2012 to complete two post-graduate degrees (Magister and Doctorat es Sciences Vétérinaires). He has been a lecturer in the Department of Veterinary Sciences for over ten years.

Project leader for several national and international programmes (PRFU 2021; PNR 2022 and RISE H2020 CANLEISH: 101007653), Dr Zeroual Fayçal attaches great importance to scientific research and educational and practical training. The director of several doctoral theses, he is also the author of several scientific articles.

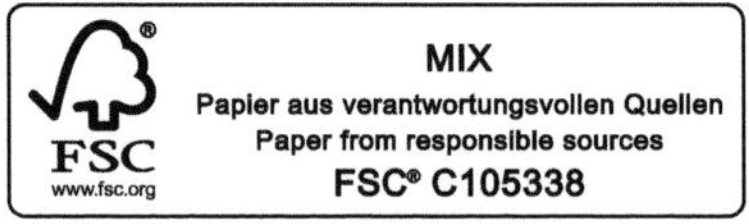

Printed by Books on Demand GmbH, Norderstedt / Germany